BANISH
YOUR
BELLY, BUTT & THIGHS
FOREVER!

BANISH

YOUR
BELLY, BUTT & THIGHS

FOREVER!

THE *REAL* WOMAN'S
GUIDE TO BODY SHAPING
& WEIGHT LOSS

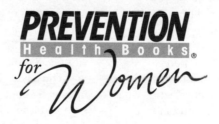

This edition first published in the UK in 2003 by
Rodale Ltd
7–10 Chandos Street
London W1G 9AD
www.rodale.co.uk

© 2000 Rodale Inc.

Illustrations © 2000 Karen Kuchar

All interior photos Mitch Mandel

Printed and bound in the UK by The Bath Press using acid-free paper from sustainable sources
3 5 7 9 8 6 4

'Customise Your Walking Technique' on page 212 was reproduced with permission of IDEA, The Health and Fitness Source, www.IDEAfit.com

A CIP record for this book is available from the British Library
ISBN 1–405–00666–8

This paperback edition distributed to the book trade by Pan Macmillan Ltd

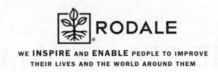

RODALE

WE **INSPIRE** AND **ENABLE** PEOPLE TO IMPROVE
THEIR LIVES AND THE WORLD AROUND THEM

About *Prevention* Health Books for Women

The editors of *Prevention* Health Books for Women are dedicated to providing you with authoritative, trustworthy, and innovative advice for a healthy active lifestyle. In all of our books, our goal is to keep you thoroughly informed about the latest breakthroughs in natural healing, medical research, alternative health, herbs, nutrition, fitness and weight loss. We cut through the confusion of today's conflicting health reports to deliver clear, concise and definitive health information that you can trust. And we explain in practical terms what each new breakthrough means to you, so you can take practical steps to improve your health and well-being.

Every recommendation in *Prevention* Health Books for Women is based upon interviews with highly qualified health authorities, including medical doctors and practitioners of alternative medicine.

Prevention Health Books for Women are thoroughly fact checked for accuracy, and we make every effort to verify recommendations, dosages and cautions.

The advice in this book will help keep you well-informed about your personal choices in health care – to help you lead a happier, healthier and longer life.

EDITOR: Sharon Faelten
CONTRIBUTING WRITERS: Donna Raskin; Kristine Napier, R.D.;
Kim Galeaz, R.D.; Roberta Duyff, R.D.;
Elizabeth Ward, R.D.; Betsy Bates;
Judith Lin Eftekhar; Susan Huxley;
Larry Keller
UK EDITOR: Esther Jagger
UK INTERIOR DESIGNER: Studio Cactus
PHOTO EDITOR: James A. Gallucci
COVER PHOTOGRAPHER: Mitch Mandel
ILLUSTRATOR: Karen Kuchar
ASSISTANT RESEARCH MANAGER: Anita C. Small
BOOK PROJECT RESEARCHER: Teresa A. Yeykal
EDITORIAL RESEARCHERS: Molly Donaldson Brown,
Lori Davis, Christine Dreisbach,
Bella Hebrew, Mary Kittel,
Elizabeth B. Price, Staci Sander,
Elizabeth Shimer, Lucille Uhlman,
Nancy Zelko
SENIOR COPY EDITOR: Amy K. Kovalski
PRODUCTION EDITOR: Cindy Updegrove
UK COVER DESIGNER: Button Design Company
LAYOUT DESIGNER: Keith Biery
ASSOCIATE STUDIO MANAGER: Thomas P. Aczel
MANUFACTURING COORDINATORS: Brenda Miller, Jodi Schaffer,
Patrick T. Smith

Rodale Healthy Living Books

VICE PRESIDENT AND PUBLISHER: Brian Carnahan
VICE PRESIDENT AND EDITORIAL DIRECTOR: Debora T. Yost
EDITORIAL DIRECTOR: Michael Ward
VICE PRESIDENT AND MARKETING DIRECTOR: Karen Arbegast
PRODUCT MARKETING MANAGER: Tania Attanasio
BOOK MANUFACTURING DIRECTOR: Helen Clogston
MANUFACTURING MANAGERS: Eileen Bauder, Mark Krahforst
RESEARCH MANAGER: Ann Gossy Yermish
COPY MANAGER: Lisa D. Andruscavage
PRODUCTION MANAGER: Robert V. Anderson Jr.
OFFICE MANAGER: Jacqueline Dornblaser
OFFICE STAFF: Suzanne Lynch Holderman, Julie Kehs,
Mary Lou Stephen, Catherine E. Strouse

CONTENTS

FOREWORD

Throw away those dowdy oversize T-shirts and tracksuits. *Banish Your Belly, Butt & Thighs Forever!* offers a comprehensive programme that shows you how to flatten your belly, trim your thighs and firm your behind so you can stop hiding behind layers of baggy clothes – forever.

As fitness editor of *Prevention* magazine, the world's largest circulation health magazine, every day I hear from women who, like you, want to target these trouble spots. Even women who aren't overweight want to get rid of that spare tyre around their middles or tone jiggly thighs or sagging butts. Now you can! The authors talked to leading weight-loss, nutrition and fitness experts to develop a plan that will take you from your first walk round the block to your final walk through the shopping mall for a new wardrobe in a smaller size. Whether this is your 1st or 50th attempt at losing weight, *Banish Your Belly, Butt & Thighs Forever!* tells you everything you need to know to go from fat to fabulous.

Here are some comments from real women who tried this programme and loved it.

- 'I can't believe what a difference such a simple programme has made. And I never felt like I was on a diet!' says Janine Slaughter, aged 37.

- 'I have tons of energy! And my husband keeps commenting on how skinny I'm getting,' says Laura Kaplus, aged 32.

- 'The exercises are straightforward and simple to do thanks to the photos, and they work,' says Brooke Myers, aged 31.

What makes this programme so successful is that you can customise it to meet your needs. If all the exercise you get is pushing a trolley round the supermarket, you can start with the low-intensity, beginner's workouts. That way, you'll avoid one of the most common beginners' mistakes – doing too much too soon – which can leave you with injuries or hating exercise.

If you're exercising regularly now but aren't satisfied with your progress, start with the high-intensity workouts for experienced exercisers. Plus, you'll discover numerous fun ways to exercise – everything from cycling to water aerobics – that target your specific trouble spots.

No weight-loss programme would be complete without a healthy diet. But this book gives you more than a 'one-size-fits-all' meal plan. The Best and Worst Body-Shaping Foods chapter can help you draw up a shopping list of low-fat, tasty foods that will help you to shed pounds. Stock up on the best ones, and you'll never feel hungry again. Best of all, you have the freedom to indulge. Even chocoholics can indulge their pleasure. What's more, you can eat out without blowing your diet. Expert dietitians show you how.

Most important, you'll feel good while you lose weight – you'll learn how to set the right goals for success and how to incorporate strategies to help you stick with your exercise programme. After years of coaching women, I know that you can't slim down if you don't feel good about yourself.

Turn the page and watch your trouble spots disappear.

Michelle Stanten

Fitness Editor
Prevention magazine

ACKNOWLEDGMENTS

Special thanks to Marjorie Albohm, an exercise physiologist, certified athletic trainer and director of sports medicine at Kendrick Memorial Hospital in Mooresville, Indiana, for developing the Body-Shaping Workouts for this programme.

Thanks also to the following registered dietitians for creating and writing the Eating Lean portion of this programme.

Kristine Napier, R.D., a registered dietitian and nutrition consultant in Mayfield Village, Ohio; consultant director of the Nutrition Enhancement Project at the Cleveland Clinic Heart Center, Preventive Cardiology Program; and author of *Power Nutrition for Chronic Illness*.

Kim Galeaz, R.D., a registered dietitian and food and nutrition consultant in Indianapolis.

Roberta Duyff, R.D., a registered dietitian and food and nutrition consultant in St Louis, Missouri, and author of *The American Dietetic Association's Complete Food and Nutrition Guide*, among other books.

Elizabeth Ward, R.D., a registered dietitian and nutrition consultant in Stoneham, Massachusetts, spokesperson for the American Dietetic Association, and author of *Pregnancy Nutrition: Good Health for You and Your Baby*, among other publications.

PART ONE

The Art of Body Shaping

Chapter 1

It's a Lifestyle, Not a Diet

It's an all too familiar experience: you take your favourite jeans out of the tumble drier, and you can't zip them up. You reckon the drier shrank them. The next morning you get dressed for work, and you can't button your skirt. That night, you get your favourite dress out of the wardrobe and it pulls across your backside.

You've gained weight. Again. The last diet you tried worked, but you've regained all the weight. Worse, it's settled just where you least want the extra curves – on your belly, butt and thighs.

If you're unhappy with your physique, you have lots of company. No doubt you've read the headlines proclaiming that more than half of the UK population over the age of 20 is overweight, and that nearly one out of every five people is clinically obese. Despite our obsession with getting thinner, more women (and men) are overweight.

Fad diets don't seem to be helping. We spend a fortune each year on weight-loss treatments, primarily diets and dietary foods. We buy diet books that claim to be the next miracle or revolution with the zeal of a chocoholic attacking a family-size bar of fruit and nut. We try high-protein diets, cabbage soup diets – even chewing gum diets.

Still, the incidence of obesity is rising rapidly and it's the same picture in many other parts of the world, particularly in the USA. Trends seem to indicate that we will see a worldwide expansion of waistlines, hips and thighs rivalling global warming in scope.

It's Not Your Fault

Much of this extra weight comes from supersize portions and mega meals. Everything from chocolate bars to breakfast cereals now comes in bigger packages than in the past. Portions in many family-type restaurants have become gargantuan. Indeed, the average 'serving' per order could sometimes feed an entire family.

'There is enormous commercial pressure for people to eat more,' says Dr Marion Nestle of the department of nutrition and food studies at New York University. 'Food companies are competing in two ways. They want you to eat their product instead of somebody else's. And they want you to eat more. It's good for business.' The obvious solution? 'Eat less,' says Dr Nestle. 'Train yourself to stop eating when you feel full. You need to be vigilant.'

Granted, this is easier said than done. But it can be done. Dr Nestle and several of her colleagues have begun practising what they preach by eating smaller portions at meals. 'The pounds just fall off,' she says. 'We're astounded.'

Developing a general knowledge of the fat and calorie content of foods is useful for planning what to eat, but don't measure and weigh your food to the point of obsession.

If you eat out, calorie counting is impossible because you don't see how the food is prepared, explains Dr Nestle. She cites an experiment in which she and several other nutritionists were taken to lunch by a newspaper reporter who asked them to estimate the number of calories and grams of fat in what they ate.

'We couldn't do it,' she says. 'We didn't even come close. It was inconceivable to me that the food we were eating had as much fat and calories as it turned out to have.'

Why Dieting Doesn't Work

There are lots of things you can – and should – do, however, in the fight against fat. In Part Two, Eating Lean, you'll learn how to shop for the right kind of food prepared in weight-friendly ways and substitute foods that are kind to your waistline and hips. Add new, healthier foods to your repertoire. Keep a food diary. Eat more fibre. Eat small meals throughout the day. You'll find out that you don't need to deny yourself the occasional biscuit or piece of chocolate – just set limits for yourself and stick to them.

In fact, you don't have to limit yourself to cabbage soup or other unusual foods to lose weight. There is no hard evidence that anybody benefits from dieting per se. In fact, 90–95 per cent of women who attempt to lose weight via dieting fail. Emerging data suggests that when women diet and then begin to lose and regain weight over and over again, the process may be driving their bodies' natural set point for weight upwards. Also, this so-called yo-yo dieting can lead to frustration and overeating.

The real weight-loss experts are women just like you who worked out how to pare pounds and pinch inches painlessly. Take Cindi Arvanites, who changed the way she cooked meals – and improved her figure in the process. By substituting lower-fat ingredients for high-fat ones or using less of the latter and eating smaller portions, Cindi has eaten more healthily and lost weight at the same time. Yet she still adds some 'calorific luxuries,' such as butter, to her recipes – just less of it. In Chapter 7 you'll find out how to do all that yourself.

Being Active Made Easy

Monitoring what you place in your mouth is half the equation. It will only work if you also burn more calories. Some of you are thinking, 'Not me.' You feel silly flouncing about in a step aerobics class with young, leotard-clad women who look like off-duty ballet dancers. Or the idea of hard exercise appeals to you about as much as 10 hours of labour pains.

But as you'll learn in this book, you don't have to train for a marathon in order to become more active. In fact, exercising can be fun. Really.

And you don't have to follow a strict regimen – unless you want to. Experts say that your chances for success are higher if you incorporate aerobic activities into your lifestyle. Take a 30-minute walk during your lunch hour, for example. Like many women, you probably associate the term *aerobic* with callisthenics done to music in a class. But technically, any sustained activity that gets your heart pumping can contribute to weight loss. And you don't have to huff and puff for hours: 30 minutes of aerobic activity most days of the week may do the trick, says Dr Laurie L. Tis of the department of kinesiology and health at Georgia State University in Atlanta.

What's more, there are dozens of ways to work exercise into your lifestyle, including but not limited to aerobics classes. Here are just a few:

- If you're a homebody, you can garden or work around the house.

- If you have teenagers, you can bicycle, skate-board, or go riding with them.

- If you're competitive, you can play table tennis, badminton, tennis or squash.

- If you like to dance, you can take up dancing. (What better way to work your abdominal muscles than belly dancing?)

- If you like to work out in the privacy of your own home, or you can't get to a gym, you can use a skipping rope, stepping or stairclimbing machine or rowing machine.

- If you have knee or back problems, you can swim.
- If you take you holidays in the Mediterranean or tropics, you can snorkel. If you are surrounded by beautiful countryside, explore it on foot.

The list goes on.

'When we talk about healthy lifestyle and quality of life issues, we're finding that it's less about that '20-minute, 75 per cent of maximum heart rate three times a week,' and more about just being generally active,' says Dr Tis. The idea is to get a minimum of 30 minutes of moderate activity in total throughout the day.

On page 182 you will meet Kate Flynn, whose story shows how a change in lifestyle can improve physique. A single mother of two, she enjoyed aerobics classes, but found it hard to make the time or shell out the money for them. Interested in keeping fit, Kate also tried running, but it hurt her knees. She didn't give up, though. Instead, she became an avid gardener who has maintained a firm body and a youthful appearance by weeding, raking, and the like.

Kate illustrates what more and more exercise and weight-loss experts are recommending: experiment with various forms of physical activity until you find one or more that you like. The advantage of doing so is that you are more likely to keep at it consistently, says Dr Charles Corbin of the department of exercise science and physical education at Arizona State University. 'The activity doesn't have to be vigorous,' he adds. If you work out about as hard as brisk walking, you can exercise for a fair amount of time without getting tired.

'When you were a kid, you enjoyed being active,' notes Dr Corbin. 'If you can find that enjoyment again, you may be much better off than if you are a member of four different health clubs, getting on treadmills all the time and doing callisthenics. It's best to find things you really enjoy.'

A Little Goes a Long Way

Still sceptical about exercise? There's a wealth of research suggesting that even modest increases in physical activity pay off.

In one study, for example, a group of 40 women who were each 33 lb (13.6 kilos) or more overweight was divided into two groups. One group did aerobic exercise for 16 weeks and ate a daily diet of 1200 calories. The other group increased their moderate-intensity physical activity by 30 minutes a day, most days of the week, while also eating a 1200-calorie diet for 16 weeks.

The first group participated in a step aerobics class, reaching a peak of 45 minutes of stepping by the eighth week. The second group was encouraged to walk rather than drive short distances, take the stairs instead of the lift, and the like. After 16 weeks, women in both groups had lost weight, but there were not significant differences between them.

In another, two-year study, 235 sedentary, overweight men and women were divided into groups similar to those in the above study. When it was over, the group that had simply begun living a more physically active lifestyle had lost slightly more weight and a greater percentage of body fat than the group that was in a structured exercise programme.

In a third study, Mayo Clinic researchers fed 16 women and men of average weight food containing 1000 calories per day above what was required to maintain their weight, and limited them to low levels of exercise. Then they measured which participants stored the most and the least amounts of the additional calories as fat.

The study volunteers gained an average of 10 lb (4.5 kilos) in two months. But those who were most active without actually exercising – they fidgeted, moved around, adjusted their posture, and so forth – gained the least weight. One volunteer burned up an average of 692 calories per day through such apparently insignificant movements. Conversely, those participants who moved around the least gained the most weight.

Finally, in yet another study more than 1000 women and men who were trying to maintain their weight were monitored for a year. Researchers found that those who spent the most time watching television gained the most weight. Among high-income women, each hour of TV viewed per day equated to an extra half-pound of weight gained over the year.

Television per se is not to blame, of course. But it's a sedentary activity. Getting up during commercial breaks to load the dishwasher or fold clothes, or taking a brief exercise break by doing jumping jacks or jogging on the spot are among the things you can do to break the lethargy cycle, says Dr Nestle.

Maybe you think vanity is a poor reason to lose weight. Fine, but your appearance isn't the only reason. Think about your health. Physically active women run less risk of dying from coronary heart disease and developing high blood pressure, colon cancer and diabetes. And all that movin' and groovin' may enhance the effect of oestrogen-replacement therapy in decreasing bone loss after the menopause.

Certainly most of us could improve on this score. While a common stereotype is that of a pot-bellied man slumped in front of the television, experts report that women are more apt to be physically inactive than men.

'But I don't have time to exercise,' you might say. Or, 'I don't have time to shop for special food – I have to eat what my family eats.'

No problem. On page 226, you'll learn how any woman, no matter how busy, can work exercise into her schedule. And in Part Two you'll discover innovative advice from dietitians who specialise in teaching women how to shop for and prepare foods that the whole family will enjoy.

You won't even know you're on a diet. Because you're not. You're living a lifestyle that puts you in control, once and for all.

Chapter 2

Your Unique Body

Three women get together for lunch. One of them, a harassed woman whose life is filled with young children and a full-time job, orders a turkey sandwich without the mayonnaise, and shows interest in the dessert menu. The oldest woman, who works part-time but is otherwise a homemaker, asks for fruit salad and cottage cheese. The youngest woman, who is single, active and loving it, hasn't eaten anything yet today and she's starving. She orders crispbread with a salad. All three of these women think they are on a diet.

Here are Margie, Sarah and Ann, three different women with one thing in common: they each want to lose weight.

- Margie, aged 40, wants to lose 20lb (9 kilos) from her hips and backside, which is the weight that she has put on since having children.
- Sarah, 52, is a career dieter. She has 30lb (13.6 kilos) to lose – weight that she's lost and regained (plus a little more) again and again.
- And finally there is Ann, 29 and single. She only has 10lb (4.5 kilos) to lose, but that weight has settled mostly on her thighs and backside within the last few years.

Do these women sound like you or your friends? They should. You see, Margie, Sarah and Ann are composites, based on what surveys reveal – and weight-loss experts confirm – to be the most common types of women dieters. Margie is the stressed-out career woman who blames her weight gain on having children. Sarah is the nurturing, sedentary, plump mother who spends an inordinate amount of time in the kitchen. Ann is the life-at-full-speed single who hardly thinks about her health.

In fact, you probably already recognise yourself – or parts of yourself – in one or more of them. And that's good, because you're going to get to know Margie, Sarah, and Ann intimately – their bodies, their eating habits, their exercise needs, their goals, their struggles. More important, you'll discover expert advice for how each can sculpt a weight-loss and body-shaping programme that is absolutely best for her. You'll learn how they can eat well, live active lives and feel better. Using them as examples, you'll be able to take advice that experts offer these women and apply it to your own efforts. If they can do it, so can you.

The Common Theme: Uniqueness

Why go through this exercise? Simple: while the major themes of weight loss are universal – eat smarter, be more active – each person needs to apply these maxims in her own way, based on the special needs of her body and circumstances.

'One of the most important considerations in weight loss is to remember that we each have a unique biochemistry, just as we each have unique fingerprints,' says Dr Michael Steelman, a weight-loss specialist in Oklahoma City. 'While there are absolute dietary and lifestyle changes we all need to make, we also have to remember that each of these changes will be unique and individual to every person.'

That means that what works for Margie isn't going to work for Ann and what works for Ann isn't going to work for Sarah. Take breakfast, for example. Margie could add a piece of fruit and replace her regular cereal with one low in sugar and high in fibre. Sarah might try having a poached egg rather than the fried eggs and sausage that her husband demands. And Ann should start eating breakfast instead of going without food until lunch.

'The basics of weight loss are really the same across the board,' says Dr Steelman. 'The "recipe" includes nutritious food, exercise, an active lifestyle and stress management. But to lose weight, each woman has to add specific ingredients in the right percentages to create the recipe that tastes just right to her palate.'

So where do you begin in building the right programme for you? By learning why you've gained weight. Like many women, Margie, Sarah and Ann have all spent a lot of time trying to lose their extra pounds, but they haven't spent any time trying to understand why they have weight problems in the first place.

To formulate a weight-loss and body-shaping plan that works for you, listen carefully to these women's stories. If you're typical of women who struggle in frustration with their weight, certain elements will mirror your experience. Do you attribute your weight gain to hormones, as Margie does? Have you been dieting your whole life and now worry about your health, like Sarah? Do you skip meals and then binge at night, like Ann? Perhaps you're a combination of all three, or just two. Whatever your situation, you're likely to find some underlying truths about why you, too, might be struggling with weight loss.

Margie: Wants to Lose Her 'Baby Fat'

At 40, Margie has two wonderful children, a demanding job, a great husband and a surplus 20lb (9 kilos) on her body. Her hips are wider than they used to be, and she hates to see her rear end in the mirror.

Margie attributes her weight gain to the hormonal changes that come with having children – along with certain lifestyle changes that come with raising children. For example, she often ends up at fast-food restaurants as she shuttles her kids between activities after school or at weekends. In order to stick to her 'diet' she tries to minimise the calorific damage by ordering small – a burger, small fries and a soft drink. Small or not, the food she orders still contributes more fat and calories than a carefully planned home-cooked meal would.

Like so many office workers, Margie also faces a constant barrage of fattening goodies at work – the leaving party chocolate cake, the birthday cream buns and the weekly-meeting croissants. Margie thinks that she does a pretty good job of limiting the damage, helping herself to just a small piece of cake.

The problem is, that isn't the only time Margie eats this kind of food. She would never tell anyone, but when she has a row with her husband or gets upset at work she'll go and buy something sweet. Sometimes it's chocolate, sometimes it's a packaged dessert, but it's always high in fat and calories. When life isn't going right for Margie, food is her best friend.

Is Having Babies Really to Blame?

Childbearing is only an excuse for being overweight. It is possible for a woman to have children without having to sacrifice her physique.

But like a lot of women, Margie is sure that having children caused her to gain weight. 'It's not true,' says Brenda Eckert, a registered dietitian in Maryland. 'Mother Nature has it set up so that if we watch our calories before and during pregnancy, during lactation and after lactation, then our weight should return to the pre-pregnancy weight.'

Margie should recognise that if she had just paid attention to the amount and types of food she ate, as well as her level of physical activity, her weight wouldn't have got out of hand, Eckert says. The weight came on because she eats high-fat, high-calorie, non-nutritious fast food with her children and because she doesn't get any exercise. Ultimately, Margie will need to deal with the underlying causes of her emotional eating, learn healthier eating patterns and become more physically active.

Sarah: The Veteran Dieter

Her four children have grown up and left home and Sarah, at 52, now works three days a week in a doctor's surgery. Her life is quiet, finally. She and her husband are happy to watch a little TV at night and see their grandchildren at weekends.

Sarah has been on every diet under the sun. She has lost and regained the same 30lb (13.6 kilos) with each of them. Of course, she never stopped cooking proper meals for her family during any of these phases. They always had eggs and bacon for breakfast and meat and potatoes for dinner. Sarah's husband likes it that way. In fact, he still likes it that way, even though he needs to lose weight too. She hates to say it, but she even overfeeds the dog, as the vet recently pointed out.

At this point in their lives, Sarah is actually beginning to worry about how the extra weight is affecting her and her husband's health. He, at least, gets some exercise from his weekly round of golf, but Sarah's hobbies are sedentary, even fattening. She likes to sew – and cook!

The Problem with Yo-Yo Thinking

Sarah's idea of a diet is to buy the latest weight-loss gimmicks, including shakes, pills and formulas. When she was younger, they worked – for a while.

Now it seems harder to lose weight, no matter what she tries. After years of losing and regaining the weight, Sarah is convinced that she has permanently broken her fat thermostat. She's sure the extra weight she has kept on since her last diet is here to stay. But here's the good news: it isn't years of yo-yo dieting that have led to Sarah's weight gain. You can't break your metabolism. 'Yes, your body composition probably changes each time you lose and regain weight,' says Eckert. 'But that doesn't mean the situation is hopeless.'

Sarah's biggest problem, says Eckert, is that she thinks of weight loss as a light switch – it's

either on or off. 'This is a sure road to failure. Sarah needs to realise that she must eat properly and be active for the rest of her life. Period.'

Nevertheless, Eckert doesn't minimise the effect Sarah's husband is having on her. 'Not getting support is hard; it's a real issue,' she says. 'Sarah is really going to have to take steps to deal with that.'

Ann: A Question of Genetics?

Ah, to be 29 and single again, Margie and Sarah think, looking longingly at Ann's slim waist and torso. What they don't realise is that, when Ann gets out of the bath and looks in the mirror, she focuses on her thighs. And when she thinks about what to order for lunch, she's thinking about her thighs. And her mother's thighs. And her sister's thighs. Ann is convinced that genetics is a curse. She has beautiful jet black hair and lovely skin – also inherited from her mother – but she's also 10lb (4.5 kilos) heavier than she was five years ago. Hidden under a sarong skirt, Ann's thighs may not be obvious to Margie and Sarah. But Ann thinks about them enough to keep them hidden.

Ann always skips breakfast and often skimps at lunch. By dinnertime, she's ravenous. And most nights she's out, discovering a new restaurant with her friends. She eats pretty sensibly then, she thinks: grilled fish, or pasta with pesto, or sweet-and-sour prawn and broccoli with a vegetable (not meat) spring roll. And, she limits herself to a glass or two of wine.

Ann used to run regularly, but her job keeps her too busy to jog on weekdays any more. Her gym membership lapsed about three months ago, and she can't remember the last time she lifted a weight. She tries to get out for a run on Sundays, though. And she often fits in a game of tennis or a swim on Saturdays.

Ann's 3000-Calorie Meal

How can someone gain weight when she's only eating one big meal a day? Pretty easily, says Eckert. 'First of all, Ann is eating more fat and calories than she realises,' she explains. Pesto and even fish (if it is grilled with butter) are brimming with fat. And restaurant portions are often larger than a 'regular', healthy serving. Add it up, and what Ann considers to be a sensible meal is landing her a full day's quota of calories – and then some.

'Plus, Ann is slowing down her metabolism by starving herself the rest of the day,' says Eckert. 'This mindset of starvation–binge, starvation–binge is a big problem.' Indeed, Ann is breaking almost every principle of sound eating. She must learn to eat reasonable portions of less fatty food, distributed throughout the day. She doesn't have the discipline – yet – of a grown-up eater.

Finally, Ann's exercise doesn't do her enough good. She may burn a few extra calories, but not nearly enough to compensate for the extra calories she consumes during the week.

The Hidden Problem (and the Real Solution)

Even though Margie, Sarah and Ann think they have nothing in common, they do. They all see their extra weight as a problem caused by some external force – the family, the failure of diets or the legacy of genetics. The reality, however, is that they are each fully responsible for the extra weight. It's their own habits that have created the problem. And it's changing their habits that will save them.

'All three of these women need to take the focus off what they think caused the weight gain and begin to look at realistic ways to change their daily lives in order to lose weight and live healthier lives,' says Terry Passano, a registered dietitian in Maryland.

For example, Margie is going to have to keep low-calorie snacks on hand for herself and her kids while they're driving to music lessons and sports matches. Or she's going to have to order grilled chicken and a salad, skip the fries and pass up dessert when they go to a fast-food restaurant.

'Each of these women has options and lots of things going for her that will help make her weight loss successful,' Passano says. 'It's great, for instance, that Sarah loves to cook. Now she just has to get used to experimenting with healthier recipes and making subtle changes in her old ones, such as switching to low-fat cheese. The whole family may actually enjoy the new, healthier meals.'

Learning by Example

How much weight do *you* want to lose? Ten pounds? Thirty? A hundred? Do you carry your extra weight on your stomach? Your backside? Your hips and thighs? Or all over?

Do you credit (or blame) heredity for your figure? Childbearing? The menopause? Do you realise all too well that you need to exercise, but hate the idea of getting all sweaty? Or just can't imagine where you'd find the time?

Do you feel that buying and preparing meals for others – your husband or children – limits your food choices to what they're willing to eat?

Even if you don't identify with every aspect of Margie's, Sarah's and Ann's approaches to dieting, the chances are you can understand the principles at work – and learn to apply them to your own circumstances.

Using Margie, Sarah and Ann as examples, the following chapters will help you with:

- How to allow for (or discount) the effects of ageing, pregnancy, the menopause and other hormonal factors on your weight and shape

- How to eat the proper number of calories for your body type and energy level

- How much dietary fat will make you feel full, and how much dietary fat will make you fat

- How to fit regular exercise into your schedule

Once you've assessed your situation you can use the meal plans, cooking techniques, food tables, exercise programmes and self-coaching tips that follow to achieve your personal weight-loss and body-shaping goals – once and for all.

Chapter 3

What You Can and Cannot Change

Margie believes that her two pregnancies have left her heavy forever. Sarah believes that the menopause – combined with a lifetime of dieting – has ruined her chances of ever being thin again. And Ann believes that her thighs are a genetic inheritance over which she has no control. Are they right?

Well, yes and no. The women's beliefs are, for the most part, half-truths. The whole truth encompasses two realities: biology plays a role in our size and shape, but we determine how much of a toll it will ultimately take. While pregnancy, dieting and genetics do play a significant role in what we weigh and how we look, our lifestyles and eating habits are even more important.

'At 20, you usually have the body you were born with, but at 40 or 60 you have a body that reflects the way you lived your life,' says Edith Hogan, a registered dietitian in Washington, DC and spokesperson for the American Dietetic Association. 'One key to successful weight loss is learning to work with, not against, who you are and what you've been given. Some things you can change, and some you can't.'

The Hormone Connection

Before we explore the details of Margie's, Sarah's and Ann's diets, we need to understand a little about the science of body shape. While calories, fat and energy expenditure determine to a great extent how much weight you'll gain throughout your life, one other factor appears in the equation – hormones.

Hormones are naturally occurring chemicals that circulate throughout our bodies. Their job is to carry a message from one organ of the body to another, influencing how the second organ will behave. In women, for example, the ovaries secrete oestrogen and progesterone, reproductive hormones that play a big role in pregnancy, breast development and 400 other bodily functions – including fat storage. They also produce testosterone and dehydroepiandrosterone (DHEA), albeit in much smaller amounts than men generate.

To a degree, hormones influence our weight and shape. Most women, for that matter, already know that menstruation, pregnancy and the menopause are hormone-related and often result in weight changes. Until recent years, many doctors (and women) thought that changes caused by hormones were a *fait accompli*. Everyone assumed that we had very little power over our body types, our fat storage and our life cycles.

That thinking has changed. Research shows that the way we eat, our activity levels and our ability to handle stress all affect our hormones – and, in turn, our hormones will affect our weight and body shape, says Dr Elizabeth Lee Vliet, founder and medical director of HER Place women's health centres in Texas, and author of *Screaming to Be Heard: Hormonal Connections Women Suspect and Doctors Ignore*. Margie, Sarah and Ann – and women like them – can learn how to help their bodies handle hormonal changes over the years.

Margie: Pregnancy, Cellulite – and Winter

Three things about her weight bug Margie. First, after each of her two pregnancies she retained 10lb extra (4.5 kilos). Second, she always gains about 7lb (3.2 kilos) in winter, bringing her total close to 30lb extra (13.6 kilos) for six months of the year. Third, Margie has cellulite, and it keeps her from wearing shorts in the summer, even though she's not quite as heavy then.

Margie assumes that these weight changes are inevitable. After all, most women are heavier after they've had a couple of babies – and everyone seems to gain weight in winter. A lot of her friends have cellulite, too, and she doubts that creams sold in department stores will help. Margie wants to eat well and exercise, but she thinks her particular problems have no solutions.

Here's what she needs to know.

Pregnancy. If a woman is at her correct weight, doctors recommend that she gain between 25 and 35lb (11–16 kilos) during her pregnancy, to support and nurture her developing child. Underweight women should gain between 28 and 40lb (13–18 kilos), while overweight women are advised to gain between 15 and 25lb (7–11 kilos). No matter how heavy she is, a woman should never diet while she's pregnant except under the guidance of a doctor.

Of 30lb (14 kilos) gained during pregnancy, for example, only 7 of those pounds (3 kilos) are comprised of fat. Amniotic fluid, other tissues and the baby itself make up the rest and are lost during the birth. So a new mother should only have a few pounds to lose after her baby is born. Women will also notice changes in the shape of their breasts (especially if they breastfeed) and belly. Likewise, their hips may also widen a bit just before birth. These changes aren't due to fat accumulation, but to alterations in the tissues and bones during pregnancy and lactation.

What Margie – and you – can change: if you retain any more than 4lb extra (2 kilos) for more than a year or two after giving birth, it's due to your diet and lifestyle, and not due to the pregnancy, says Edith Hogan. Most women should be able to get back to, or just above, their pre-pregnancy weight.

While you can't change the actual shape of your breast tissue, weight training can give your breasts a little more lift by increasing the strength of your pectoral, or chest, muscles. Extra folds of skin can't be exercised off, but losing unwanted fat through diet and exercise can get rid of tummy rolls. Hips that widened to accommodate pregnancy cannot be changed, unless the extra width is from a layer of fat. (If you can pinch it, it's fat.)

Cellulite. Although cellulite looks different from other fat, it really isn't. It looks dimpled because of the way the fat is connected to the muscle underneath – strands of connective tissue pull tight where the fat is thickest (usually on the hips, buttocks and thighs). Not everyone who has a lot of body fat has cellulite, and conversely, some otherwise slender women do have cellulite. The tendency to develop cellulite seems to have a lot to do with genetics and age, says Dr Vliet. Women are more prone to cellulite than men, presumably because of a gender-linked predisposition to gain weight on the hips, buttocks and thighs.

What Margie – and you – can change: you can certainly change the amount of fat on your body. This book shows you how. And when you reduce the amount of fat, you'll reduce the appearance of cellulite. If, however, you lose excess body fat but what remains is still in the form of cellulite, over-the-counter products and exercise may temporarily help to improve its appearance, says Dr Vliet. But no cream or beauty salon treatment will actually get rid of cellulite. She adds that cutting down on processed foods, which tend to be higher in fat and salt, and soft drinks as well as increasing your water intake and exercise may diminish your risk of developing cellulite in the first place.

Winter weight gain. During cold winter months, almost everyone gains weight. For one thing, we tend to be less active then, says Dr

Three Women, Three Body Types

If you're like a lot of women, you can probably identify with Margie, Sarah or Ann. We may vary in age, weight and height, but we tend to carry extra weight in three different areas, which are shown here.

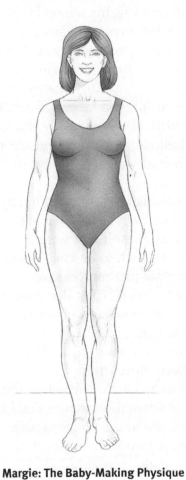 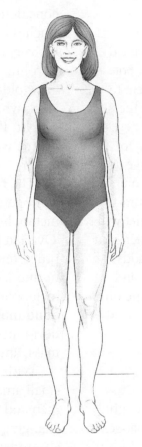 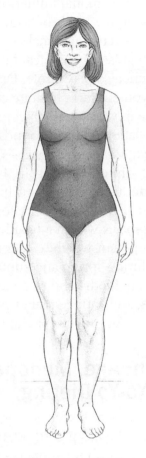

Margie: The Baby-Making Physique

Having children changes the shape of your hips and belly (especially if you deliver by caesarean section) and usually adds a couple of pounds to your weight. Of the three body types this is the easiest to change, since controlling your weight before pregnancy and after can help prevent pregnancy-induced weight accumulation after having one or more children.

Sarah: The Apple-Shaped Physique

Post menopausal women like Sarah are likely to become apple-shaped, since hormonal changes prompt their bodies to store fat around their abdominal organs. Because intra-abdominal fat carries greater health risks than lower-body fat, it's best to minimise weight gain here even if appearance isn't an issue for you.

Ann: The Pear-Shaped Physique

For women who are years away from the menopause, like Ann, most body weight settles below the abdomen on the thighs, buttocks and hips. Of the three body types, this is the most challenging to trim — but it can be done.

Vliet. But hormones also play a part. Less sunlight means that our bodies produce more melatonin, a hormone that regulates our sleep–wake cycles. 'Like bears, we "hibernate" to some degree,' Dr Vliet explains. 'But remember, part of the bear's ability to hibernate depends on its ability to store fat, which is helped by melatonin.'

Other hormonal influences, such as a decrease in the levels of both oestradiol (a naturally occurring female hormone) and a mood-regulating chemical in the brain called serotonin, also play a role, Dr Vliet says. For some women, carbohydrate cravings seem to increase in winter, which contributes to the accumulation of extra pounds.

What Margie – and you – can change: To prevent winter weight gain, fight the urge to stay indoors, says Dr Vliet. Instead, get out and exercise. 'Eating high-fibre foods and numerous smaller meals within a healthy winter diet will also keep your weight closer to that which you enjoy during spring and summer,' she adds. High-fibre foods tend to be lower in fat and calories, and eating smaller portions more often increases your metabolic rate.

Sarah: Age, Menopause and Yo-Yo Dieting

Sarah has spent her life struggling with weight. Now that she has passed 50, the latest changes in her figure are all the more discouraging. With the menopause, her body has morphed from a generous hourglass shape to a round apple, and she feels flabbier than ever.

Meanwhile, the idea of another diet is enough to send her running. And rightly so. 'Sarah's metabolism has most likely slowed down in response to her years of dieting and being inactive,' says dietitian Brenda Eckert, 'Another episode of simply cutting down on calories won't help Sarah lose weight any more. Her age and history of inappropriate dieting will work against her.'

Does that mean Sarah has to give up?

Absolutely not. She just has to do things differently this time. Here's what Sarah and women like her need to consider.

Ageing and the menopause. At one time, doctors thought there was nothing women (or men) could do to fight the ageing process – bellies got bigger, muscles went flabby, and everyone ate less but gained more weight.

Now, the effects of ageing are no longer considered inevitable, says Dr Diana Dell, who teaches obstetrics and gynaecology at the Duke University Medical Center in Durham, North Carolina. 'The things that really change as you grow older are your muscle mass and activity level, which in turn affect your body shape and weight. If you build and maintain muscle and stay active, then your weight won't change very much.'

The hormonal changes that accompany menopause do, however, affect a woman's metabolism and, as a result, her weight. 'Ovarian hormones, such as oestrogen and progesterone, are not just reproductive hormones,' says Dr Vliet. 'They also have a metabolic role in the body and help you to build muscle and bone. So when these hormones decline, so do muscle and bone mass, and the body stores more fat.'

With the drop in female hormones, the small amounts of adrenal hormones that both men and women produce come into play, changing a more feminine, hourglass figure into a rounder, more 'male', physique.

Hormones can be readjusted with HRT (hormone-replacement therapy), but never attempt to do so without consulting your doctor. Oestrogen-replacement products that supply oestradiol can help to prevent muscle and bone loss as well as the weight gain associated with the menopause, says Dr Vliet. Progesterone, on the other hand, promotes weight gain and is often combined with oestrogen, for various reasons. Oestrogen-like compounds found in some plants, such as soya, may contribute to weight distribution and the maintenance of a healthy female body shape.

What Sarah – and you – can change: Regardless of whether you take some form of HRT, if you overeat and don't exercise you won't slim down or shape up. It's a simple rule – energy begets energy. If you ask your muscles and bones to move, they'll stimulate the process of using fat for fuel.

The solution is to do activities that are aerobic (such as walking) and weight-bearing (also walking and strength training), says Dr Vliet. Both of these activities will mimic what a youthful body contributes to metabolism.

Yo-yo dieting. Repeated weight loss and gain changes the structure and number of your fat cells, which can ultimately make it much easier for you to regain weight you've worked hard to lose. Fat cells first increase in size during a weight-gain period, but when they reach their maximum size, they divide, creating two fat cells from one. Once created, fat cells never disappear; they can only shrink.

What Sarah – and you – can change: As Sarah and other yo-yo dieters have discovered, repeated weight loss and gain makes it increasingly difficult to lose weight, because they end up with more fat cells than when they started. Still, fat cells will always be able to change size – to grow or shrink – so losing weight is not impossible.

'This time around, Sarah needs to focus on her lifetime plan to keep weight off, not just her short-term diet to lose weight quickly,' says weight-loss specialist Dr Michael Steelman.

Experts agree that exercise keeps weight from returning – and exercise is exactly what was missing from Sarah's past efforts.

Ann: PMS, Body Shape and Heredity

Despite usually staying within 10lb (4.5 kilos) of her goal weight, Ann is plagued by a week of PMS every month that temporarily adds another few pounds to her frame. She feels so bloated and fat that she has accumulated a second, larger wardrobe for these days, which help Ann feel more comfortable at a time when she's already prone to crying.

But two other things bother Ann even more than her premenstrual weight gain. She harbours a secret that both embarrasses and frightens her: her mother is more than 100lb (45 kilos) overweight. So even though Ann only has 10lb (4.5 kilos) to lose now, to her they're a sign of what's to come. She already has cellulite on her thighs and her body is quite pear-shaped. She obsesses about her weight and 'heavy thighs' and feels doomed to follow in her mother's footsteps.

Ann's worries are valid, but her situation isn't hopeless. Here's where she stands.

Premenstrual bloating. Seven to 10 days before their period, most women gain a few pounds because of water retention. Progesterone levels instigate these temporary weight gains that disappear once the period starts. It's a natural part of the reproductive cycle, although not all women experience bloating and other premenstrual symptoms.

What Ann – and you – can change: a few simple changes can minimise premenstrual bloating, says Dr Vliet. She recommends reducing water retention by cutting some salt from your diet, increasing your activity level, eating more fibre, and consuming more magnesium, a mineral that plays a role in fluid balance. 'Our lifestyles play a large role in whether or not the changes that come along with our menstrual cycles will be positive or negative,' she says. If problems persist, Dr Vliet recommends having your hormone levels checked.

If you've consistently gained an extra pound or two *after* your period, you've been eating too much before and during your period.

Pears and apples. Women tend to accumulate fat in two ways – in the shape of pears or apples.

Like Ann, most women are pears until middle age. 'Your body shape changes as you grow older because of the hormonal changes that occur as the years go by,' Dr Vliet explains. 'After menopause, we produce less oestrogen and progesterone, and that causes us to begin to gain weight the way men do, over the tummy.' This is due to the relative excess of testosterone and DHEA as oestradiol declines, she says.

Ann believes that all the extra calories from her late-night food fests accumulate on her thighs. The truth is that the first few pounds might head to her lower body, but the rest distribute themselves all over. 'Everyone has a particular pattern of weight gain,' says Dr Steelman. 'You can't control or change those genes, but no one gains weight in just one place.'

What Ann – and you – can change: whether you're trying to prevent flabby thighs when you're young or head off a bountiful belly when you're older, the best strategy is not to gain weight in the first place. If, like Ann, you've already accumulated a few extra pounds, you can still influence the shape of your lower body with resistance training and abdominal exercises – if you also keep the fat off through diet and exercise, says Rick Kahley, an exercise physiologist and personal trainer in Georgia.

Genetics. Ann is obviously aware that genetics plays a significant role in body weight. If you have two obese parents (meaning that they weigh at least 20 per cent more than they should), the risk that you will be obese is about 80 per cent. If, like Ann, one of your parents is obese, your risk is 23 per cent. If neither of your parents is obese, you have a less than 10 per cent risk of being obese. Likewise, some families or ethnic groups have a genetic tendency to gain weight or, conversely, have a high basal metabolic rate.

Two factors seem to be involved in heredity and weight gain. First, scientists have identified a gene (called the obese gene) that is responsible for leptin, a hormone that lets you know that you're full and can stop eating. Researchers believe that in some people this gene doesn't work properly, and their cell receptors don't receive, or can't recognise, signals that help them stop eating.

For relatively few women, the second possible factor is adaptation. Until the twentieth century, food wasn't plentiful for many human beings. So historically, our bodies have learned to store what they get to make sure they still have energy available when food is scarce. Over the course of several generations, some ethnic groups have become more adept than others at storing food as fat, in order to protect against times of famine, says Dr Vliet.

What Ann – and you – can change: it takes work to fight your genes, but it can be done. 'If Ann commits herself to staying in good physical shape, then she won't gain the fat that she's afraid of,' says Grace Mello, a registered dietitian in Rhode Island. 'Ann and her sisters and parents may share the same basic shape. But if one works out regularly and eats well and the others don't, you will see a difference in their figures.'

Biology Is Not Destiny

Margie's, Sarah's and Ann's concerns are all legitimate. And, yes, hormones and our genetic backgrounds do influence our size and shape. We can't change our height, our sex or the basic chemistry of our bodies, but we have a lot of control over our weight.

'The best thing anyone can do is commit themselves to habits that research has shown lead to weight loss and weight maintenance,' says Brenda Eckert. 'People who have been successful at weight loss tend to have a positive outlook on their food intake and exercise habits, weigh themselves about three times a week, exercise consistently and keep a record of what they eat and their activity.'

Why do these things work? Because many overweight people don't accurately relate how much they eat and how little they exercise. 'Behaviour and habits are really the deciding factors for most people regarding weight,' says Edith Hogan. 'The eating, exercise and attitude habits you practise throughout your life have much more of an impact on your weight than genetics.'

PART TWO

Eating Lean

Chapter 4

Ten Winning Principles of Eating Lean

Stop treating food as the enemy! You can't live without it, so you might as well make peace with it. And the sooner you accept that no foods are inherently bad and that you can enjoy a rich and rewarding relationship with food, the sooner your battle against excess weight will be won.

Of course, weight loss doesn't just happen. You need a plan – and a set of guiding principles. Below are 10 that weight-loss experts swear by.

Keep in mind that for results to be permanent, you have to lose weight *your* way. What put your best friend into size 12 jeans won't necessarily do the trick for you. So mould the following principles into a programme that you can actually enjoy – and stick with.

1. Take stock of what you're eating now. You say you don't understand why those extra pounds cling to your body? You're eating low-fat, getting lots of fruit and vegetables, avoiding empty calories (high-calorie food with little or no nutritional value) and choosing foods high in nutrients like iron and calcium. Or are you? The only way you'll really know is to write down what you eat. Don't groan! A food diary is an effective weight-loss tool. Keep one for at least three days.

2. Shop smart. You have to eat to lose weight! The trick is to eat differently from how you eat now. The easiest way is to become a smart shopper. Simple substitutions will let you cut calories and grams of fat without missing them.

3. Balance your fat intake. Obsessing about each and every gram of fat isn't the goal. The goal is awareness of fat in foods so you can learn to balance high-fat with low-fat. There's room in every diet for high-fat foods. But you have to know which foods do have more fat so you can plan to eat less of those.

4. Learn the difference between hunger and thirst. People often think they're hungry when they're actually thirsty. Try drinking a glass of cold water when the urge to nibble hits. Then see if your hunger disappears after a few minutes. Water gives you a sense of fullness so learn to love it.

5. Fill up on fibre. Fibre's not sexy, but it can help you fit into that slinky little red dress. That's because, logically enough, high-fibre foods are filling and so prevent you from overeating. Fibre-rich foods take up more space in your stomach, so you feel satisfied longer.

How much fibre do you need? Meat eaters get about 23g a day, vegetarians between 40 and 50. Aim somewhere between the two for general health as well as cancer prevention, though the full 50g will do you no harm. Fruit, vegetables, dried beans, cereals and wholegrain breads contain plenty of fibre.

6. Eat all day long. That's music to a weight-watcher's ears! Most weight-loss experts now agree that eating small meals more frequently throughout the day really keeps you satisfied – and prevents binges later in the evening. When people front-load their calories (by eating earlier in the day) and then eat every three to four hours, they appease their appetites. If you don't honour your day

Why You Crave Fat

Think of it as nature's cruel joke. Your brain is actually programmed to crave fat. In fact, there are several appetite-control chemicals in the brain that turn on your desire for fat, says registered dietitian Elizabeth Somer.

'The first of these chemicals is galanin, which is released from the hypothalamus (a gland in the brain) about midday and stays on through the evening hours,' Somer says. It entices you to choose fatty foods like pasta with cream sauce for lunch instead of chicken breast.

Ironically, if you eat too much fat at lunch, galanin escalates and makes you likely to overeat fat later in the day as well. 'So if you have a salad with lots of high-fat dressing, you're more likely to crave a big bowl of ice cream at 9 p.m.,' Somer explains. Fat cravings are also stimulated by endorphins, proteins in the brain. They make eating fat pleasurable, so you're likely to want more of that food later on.

Carbohydrates also play a role, increasing the release of serotonin in the brain, which provides a calming effect and elevates your mood. Many high-fat foods, such as cakes and biscuits, are high in carbohydrates.

Don't blame your brain entirely, though. 'Our body chemistry is geared to a time when calories could be in short supply at any turn,' says Somer. But with supermarket shelves stuffed to the gills, famine isn't likely. We just eat as if it were.

There are two more causes of fat cravings. Hormonal fluctuations in the 10 days before a menstrual period often cause women to experience an increased desire for fatty, sugary foods. So can skipping meals. According to Somer, people who skip breakfast and eat erratically are more prone to cravings, mood swings and fatigue later in the day.

So what's the solution? 'Work with your cravings, not against them,' advises Somer. If you know that you're prone to cravings in the mid-afternoon, plan a nutritious snack that will satisfy the craving.

What if it's chocolate you lust after? Just have it! You already know what happens if you don't – you eat something else but don't feel satisfied. Then you eat something else. A bunch of calories later, you reach for the chocolate. You're far worse off than if you'd eaten the chocolate in the first place. Try to limit yourself to a few pieces of chocolate, though, or try something lighter – perhaps chunks of fresh fruit dipped in chocolate syrup.

---

appetite, you'll have a wicked evening appetite to contend with.

7. Stop eating when you're satisfied. Losing extra pounds and keeping them off will be easier once you learn to distinguish between fullness and satiety. Fullness is the weight of food in your stomach. You can feel full from 10 heads of lettuce, but will you be satisfied? Probably not, so you just keep on eating. Satiety is the level of satisfaction you get from eating. And the best way to be satisfied is to eat foods with a variety of flavours, colours and textures. Think of chicken parmigiana, baby carrots, fettuccine and a tossed salad with mixed lettuce and chopped yellow peppers.

8. Don't skip meals. Going without meals is a classic form of deprivation among career dieters. When you eliminate meals you deprive your body of adequate calories for energy, not to mention valuable disease-fighting nutrients. Skipping breakfast is a major deterrent to successful weight loss.

9. If you want it, eat it – sometimes. Deprivation doesn't work. It never has. It never will. You don't need to deprive yourself while trying to lose weight. You don't need to deprive yourself while trying to lose weight. You can still eat your favourite foods. Learn to have smaller portions and relish every bite.

10. Enjoy what you eat. Slow down! Enjoy everything you eat. Many people eat so fast that they don't actually taste the food. And because of that, they aren't really satisfied, which sets them up for overeating later on. It's a vicious circle.

Chapter 5

The Best and Worst Body-Shaping Foods

On any given day, you face dozens of food and drink choices. Eggs or a croissant? Coffee or tea? Club sandwich or soup and salad? Chicken or fish? Pizza or fish and chips? Beer or wine?

Each decision, big or small, can be part of your strategy to lose weight – and that doesn't mean living on carrot sticks and water. On the contrary, say experts, foods you've been shunning aren't forbidden at all. And some foods you thought were low-cal may be delivering hidden fat and calories.

'There really are no best or worst foods, only overall ways of eating that can be best or worst for you,' says Roberta Duyff, a food and nutrition consultant in St Louis, Missouri, and author of *The American Dietetic Association's Complete Food and Nutrition Guide*. 'You need to enjoy a variety of foods, and not too much or too little of any one food. Certainly go easy on high-calorie, high-fat foods. What counts is the fat and calories in your overall diet.' Other dietitians agree.

'All kinds of negative feelings come into play when you eat so-called bad foods,' says Kim Galeaz, a food and nutrition consultant in Indianapolis. 'Many people start to feel guilt, anxiety and remorse. I'd like everyone to get over this 'good/bad' notion and start eating for enjoyment.'

Not only are you 'allowed' to eat your favourite foods, you *should* eat them, say experts. 'It's easier to stick to a healthy eating plan when you include some favourites,' says Elizabeth Ward, a registered dietitian and nutrition consultant in Stoneham, Massachusetts, spokesperson for the American Dietetic Association, and author of *Pregnancy Nutrition: Good Health for You and Your Baby*. 'Lose your all-or-nothing dieting mentality, and gain some peace. Just because you ate more than you should at one meal doesn't spell dietary disaster. And keep in mind that you can eat more food when you include daily physical activity.'

'You don't have to limit your choices to the best in any category, or even completely avoid those in the worst,' says Kristine Napier, a registered dietitian and nutrition consultant in Ohio; consultant director of the Nutrition Enhancement Project at the Cleveland Clinic Heart Center, Preventive Cardiology Program; and author of *Power Nutrition for Chronic Illness*. The following lists should be used as they were intended – to guide you towards the better choices most of the time. '"Best" selections are exceptionally helpful when you're trying to eat just a little leaner to counteract something with more calories you ate the previous day,' adds Napier.

You can also use these examples to make trade-offs during the course of the day – a light dinner to compensate for selecting a special treat at lunch or celebrating with food at midday, for example.

BREAD, ROLLS, BAGELS AND OTHER BAKED GOODS

Remember when dieters left the bun and ate the burger? Back then, carbohydrates were the bad guys and protein was all the rage. (Sometimes, fat was the rage, too. Does the low-carbohydrate diet ring a bell? No bread, but all the bacon you wanted.)

Those fads didn't make sense then, and they still don't. True, high-protein diets help you shed a few pounds quickly – because they dehydrate your cells. That fast weight loss is nothing more than life-sustaining water being wrung out of your cells. Worse, high-protein diets may place stress on your kidneys and encourage heart disease and cancer, especially if most of the protein comes from meat and other animal foods.

While convincing people that high-protein diets were the answer, media hype bad-mouthed carbohydrates. It still comes as a surprise to many people that not all bread is fattening. In fact, if chosen properly, bread is an essential in a lifelong weight-control routine.

The carbs in wholegrain foods, including wholegrain breads, are so rich in nutrients that dietitians advise 7–10 portions daily. Wholegrains are also high in fibre. High-fibre foods fill you up but with fewer calories, alleviate hunger because they are metabolised slowly, and stop you absorbing some of the calories in the other foods you eat.

Don't confuse simple carbohydrates with complex ones, however. Complex carbs are wholegrains fruit, and vegetables. Think of them as packages, the wrapping being the fibre and the insides a wealth of vitamins, minerals,

Best and Worst Bread, Rolls, Bagels and Other Baked Goods

To qualify as healthy, bread items should have fewer than 4g of fat per ounce. Also, look for breads with at least 2g of fibre per serving.

BEST CHOICES			
Item	**Portion**	**Calories**	**Grams of Fat**
Wholegrain bread	1 slice 30g (1oz)	70	1.1
Wholemeal pitta	1 small pitta 30g (1oz)	74	0.7
Swedish-style rye bread	1 slice 30g (1oz)	65	1.0

WORST CHOICES			
Item	**Portion**	**Calories**	**Grams of Fat**
Chocolate chip muffin	1 muffin 115g (4oz)	370	15.0
Garlic bread	1 restaurant portion 100g (3½oz)	360	17.0
Croissant	1 medium 50g (2oz)	231	12.0
Seasoned croûtons	30g (1oz)	132	5.2

protective substances called phytochemicals, protein and even more fibre. Simple carbohydrates are stripped-down versions. Examples include white bread and white flour, pretzels and bagels. They're not loaded with fat, but they contain few nutrients.

Shopping Smart

For the bread you eat to qualify as the staff of life, you have to make the right choices when shopping. Here's what to look for.

Bread. Think colour. Rich and varied shades of brown are often a clue that you're getting the wholegrain. But they're not a foolproof indication. Molasses, caramel and other colouring agents can help white bread masquerade as its healthier cousin. Make sure that the label confirms your choice. Look for words like '100 per cent wholemeal.' And check that some type of wholegrain flour is listed as the first ingredient.

Providing your tastebuds with a wide variety of flavours satisfies you with fewer calories. So buy small loaves of different wholegrain breads. That way, they won't go stale before you finish them. (Alternatively, buy larger loaves and freeze part of each.)

When you cut bread, aim for 1 oz (30 gram) slices. Get your kitchen scales out, weigh your loaf and then cut it into appropriate-sized pieces. One ounce of bread counts as one serving of wholegrains.

If there's a bread machine collecting dust on your shelves, put it to use. Make your own wholegrain loaves. If using mixes, choose ones that have no more than 1g of fat but at least 2g of fibre per 100-calorie serving.

Bagels. Again, buy a variety if you can. Even more important, pay attention to bagel size. Many bakery versions are the equivalent of five slices of bread and weigh in at around 390 calories. Depending on how you want to apportion your grain servings, cut these large bagels into halves or thirds.

Rolls and fancy breads. The fancier they get, the fattier they are. Some of the worst offenders are the ready-to-bake ones. Check the labels for fat and calories. As for garlic bread – do you really want to squander 360 calories and 17g of fat (for a 3½oz portion) on an accompaniment? And *oui*, croissants can be worse still (even before you slather on the butter). Preserve them for special occasions. Try also to avoid or minimise Italian-style filled breads, pizza breads, focaccia and ciabatta. Though delicious, they tend to contain lots of oil (quite apart from the fat in any fillings).

French bread, pitta bread and muffins. These items tend to be very low in fat with a reasonable number of calories. Try to find wholemeal versions – even pittas now come in wholemeal versions. (But please avoid the temptation to fill those 'nooks and crannies' in the muffins with butter!)

Spreads to add: apple butter and fruit purées. These have little or no fat, but do contain some vitamins and fibre. Buy them from health food shops or make your own. Place stewed apples, pears, prunes, apricots or peaches in a food processor with a splash of skimmed milk and a sprinkle of ground cinnamon and brown sugar. Blend until smooth. Store in the refrigerator for up to a week.

Weight-Friendly Substitutions

Traditional Scandinavian crispbreads are easier to find than ever. Resembling thin crackers, these delightfully crispy breads are made with a combination of wheat, barley, potato and rye flours. Serve them as the Scandinavians do – with soups, salads and low-fat cheeses. They're fat-free, fibre-rich and naturally low in calories – just 104 per 1oz (30g) slice, compared to 132 for croûtons and 360 for garlic bread.

Eating Out

In some restaurants, bread baskets rival the dessert trolley. What used to be a basket of plain white bread has now become a bakery full of choices accompanied by a pat of butter. Worse, the basket arrives when you're hungriest and least able to resist it. Before you know it, you've eaten a meal-size quantity.

The best way to manage this temptation is to head it off. Ask for the butter to be removed.

You might even want the basket taken away, leaving just one piece of bread or one roll per person. If you're with friends and they want the bread to stay, choose something plain, like French bread or a breadstick. Then make sure they park the basket on their side of the table, out of your reach.

MAKE IT BETTER

Waistline-Friendly American-Style Muffins

MAKES 10–12 MUFFINS

Per muffin

119 calories

3.2g of fat

(23 per cent of calories from fat)

These muffins are great as an on-the-go breakfast. Don't confuse them with English muffins, which you split and toast. These are really small cakes (but, in this version, full of good things and low in unhealthy ingredients). To cut the fat from similar recipes of your own, use two egg whites or 60g (2oz) of fat-free egg substitute in place of each whole egg. Replace whole milk with skimmed milk, and reduce the oil to one tablespoon per 115g (4oz) of flour.

90g (3oz) unbleached plain flour	*½ teaspoon grated orange zest*
120g (6oz) wholemeal plain flour	*90ml (3fl oz) orange juice*
30g (1oz) oat bran	*1 egg white, lightly beaten*
1½ teaspoons baking powder	*2 tablespoons rapeseed oil*
½ teaspoon ground cinnamon	*2 tablespoons clear honey*
pinch of ground allspice	*1 medium carrot, grated*

Preheat the oven to 200°C/400°F/gas 6. Use a non-stick muffin tin, or line an ordinary one with silicone paper or paper cases. In a medium bowl, stir together the unbleached flour, wholemeal flour, oat bran, baking powder, cinnamon and allspice. In a small bowl, combine the orange zest, orange juice, egg white, oil and honey. Add to the flour mixture and stir until just combined. Stir in the carrot. Spoon the batter into the muffin tin, filling each cup about three-quarters full. Bake for 20 minutes, or until a skewer inserted near the centres comes out clean. Remove and cool completely on a wire rack.

To store: *individually wrap each muffin in a freezer bag and freeze until ready to serve.*

To serve: *thaw overnight at room temperature. Or thaw and reheat each muffin in a microwave oven on high power (100 per cent) for 15–20 seconds.*

BEVERAGES

When it comes to liquid calories, women who watch their weight fall into two camps.

Some can recite the fat and calorie count for hundreds of foods but don't keep track of what they drink, which can squelch their weight-control efforts like a tidal wave.

Others are well aware that a canned soft drink contains 150 calories and nearly as much sugar as two chocolate bars.

The fact is that whether the source of your calories is food or drink, if you take in more calories than your body needs you will gain weight.

Water is the one beverage that assists your weight-loss efforts. Studies show that people who drink water before meals consume fewer calories and have an easier time taking off excess pounds. That's because water fills your stomach. And when your stomach is full, you don't eat as much.

So, when used appropriately wet calories can help, not hinder, your body-shaping efforts. Here's how.

Best and Worst Beverages

From a strictly calorific standpoint, plain water is the best thing you can drink. Beverages that contain fat and sugar are the worst. If your tastebuds need excitement but your hips don't need the fat and calories, look for unsweetened beverages. Drinks that offer some nutrition in return for their calorific cost, such as an 240ml (8fl oz) glass of skimmed milk, are also a wise choice. Serving sizes given here are typical for each drink.

BEST CHOICES

Beverage	Serving Size	Calories	Grams of Fat
Still or sparkling water	240ml (8fl oz)	0	0.0
Unsweetened, flavoured water	240ml (8fl oz)	0	0.0
Unsweetened, flavoured iced tea	240ml (8fl oz)	5	0.0
Vegetable juice	240ml (8fl oz)	46	0.2
Calcium-fortified orange juice	240ml (8fl oz)	120	0.7
Grape juice	240ml (8fl oz)	127	0.2

WORST CHOICES

Beverage	Serving Size	Calories	Grams of Fat
Piña colada	240ml (8fl oz)	466	4.8
Chocolate milkshake	360ml (12fl oz)	430	13.0
Eggnog	240ml (8fl oz)	342	19.0
Cappuccino with whole milk	360ml (12fl oz)	288	10.0
Regular fizzy soft drink	360ml (12fl oz)	150	0.0
Beer	360ml (12fl oz)	146	0.0

MAKE IT BETTER

Strawberry-Banana Smoothie

MAKES 4 SERVINGS

Per serving
•
85 calories
•
0.5g fat
•
*(5 per cent calories
from fat)*

Made properly, fruit smoothies are an excellent breakfast or midday pick-me-up. In contrast, the bottled versions are sticky sweet with fruit syrup and you'll consume lots of extra calories – often in excess of 300 calories per 240ml (8fl oz) with very little nutrition to show for the calorie burst.

455g (1lb) frozen strawberries, sliced

1 large banana, sliced

120ml (4fl oz) orange juice

120ml (4fl oz) fat-free vanilla yogurt or skimmed milk

6 ice cubes

Place all the ingredients in a blender and blend until thick and smooth.

Shopping Smart

For tips on buying milk and soya milk, see Milk and Dairy on page 65. Otherwise, follow these purchasing tips.

Water. Given that water has zero fat and calories and can keep you from overeating, bottled water (still or sparkling) should appear on every supermarket list. Buy enough for a week. (If you drink tap water, fill four or five small reusable sipper bottles and chill them in the refrigerator. Then carry water with you during the day.)

Coffee and coffee drinks. True, coffee contributes only 5 calories – if you drink it black. The real damage, however, comes from speciality coffees – the lattes, mochas, cappuccinos and other tall treats sold in coffee bars and shops. Choose poorly, and you've just blown your dessert calories for the next month. An 8 fl oz (240ml) regular café mocha splashes in at 493 calories and 49g of fat. Order it with skimmed milk and sans whipped cream (substitute the foam from steaming the skimmed milk), add artificial sweetener, and sneak by with just 120 calories. You're out the door with a chocolate fix – and loads of slimming, virtuous self-esteem.

Iced tea. If you're going to drink iced tea, drink plain old-fashioned iced tea – made from tea bags or leaf tea and flavoured with lemon. It has just two calories, plus you get plenty of water into the bargain. Grab a 16 fl oz (500ml) bottle of flavoured, sweetened iced tea, and you've got the equivalent of a canned soft drink.

Juices. Juice counts towards the five daily servings of fruit and vegetables that experts recommend as rich sources of vitamins, minerals, fibre and other protective nutrients. But even unsweetened juice contains quite a lot of sugar. Two particularly helpful kinds are calcium-fortified orange juice and vegetable juice. The former helps satisfy the essential bone-building calcium requirement for women who don't drink milk. And vegetable juice offers a wide variety of nutrients for few calories (46 calories in 8fl oz /240ml).

Alcohol. Experts agree that people who drink red wine in moderation seem to enjoy some protection against heart disease. Still, if you're watching your weight that benefit comes at a price – 7 calories per gram of alcohol, or about 103 calories per 5fl oz (160ml) glass. If you drink spirits, like gin or vodka, you'll quaff about 100 calories in a measure, depending on the proof, plus those in whatever mixer you choose. Liqueurs are even higher, at 160 calories per 1½fl oz (45ml) glass. As for those tropical cocktails like piña coladas – well, you might as well be drinking a chocolate milkshake.

The other trouble with alcohol? It can erase your willpower – resulting in even more excess calories than the alcohol alone.

If you don't drink and you're watching your weight, don't start now. Both black and green tea, which have zero calories, may provide heart-protecting benefits similar to those of red wine. And if you do drink, keep the calories from alcohol to a minimum.

Weight-Friendly Substitutions

If you just have to have a higher-calorie beverage, try the following substitutes.

- Instead of regular lemonade (99 calories per 8fl oz/240ml), substitute artificially sweetened lemonade drink (5 calories).
- Instead of wine (103 calories per 5fl oz/160ml), have a wine spritzer (62 calories for the same size drink).
- Instead of a chocolate milkshake (430 calories

for 12fl oz/350ml), order a café mocha made with skimmed milk, no whipped cream (120 calories for the same size).

Eating Out

A couple of beers, a glass of wine, after-dinner coffee or liqueur – extra calories can accumulate so easily when you're eating out. Managing liquid calories begins before you leave home. Enjoy a tall glass of water before you leave your home or office for a meal out. You'll consume less, starting with the bread basket.

When you do order something to drink, order fancy sparkling water with lime instead of an alcoholic drink, which can quickly erase your willpower just as you have so many scrumptious foods to choose from. If you've eaten lightly all day to save calories for a special dinner out (which is a great idea), beware: alcohol is absorbed more quickly on an empty stomach; just a little alcohol can quickly become too much.

If dinner in a restaurant just wouldn't be special without wine, order something expensive by the glass: you'll be less likely to have two or three.

CEREALS

Cold or hot, cereal is a great way to start your day. Studies show that women who skip or skimp on breakfast tend to nibble more during the mid- and late morning, perhaps eating even more calories than if they'd eaten breakfast in the first place. So eating breakfast may help you lose weight.

Of course, a breakfast of bacon and eggs won't help your weight-loss goals. Fried eggs and two rashers of bacon followed by toast with butter will gird you with about 28g of fat and 395 calories. In contrast, a bowl of bran flakes, a small glass of skimmed milk and a handful of fresh berries will supply 1g of fat and 200 calories.

Breakfast cereals are made from grains – wheat, oats, corn, barley, rice, quinoa or a multi-grain mixture. Except for some kinds of muesli, which may contain saturated vegetable fat from coconut flakes, most ready-to-eat cereals are low in calories from fat. For the most part, cereal is one of your best sources of complex carbohydrates (which, say nutrition experts, should account for 55–60 per cent of your daily calories).

Some cereals provide as much as 8–12g of

Best and Worst Cereals

Most cereals are low in fat and can also be a source of many vitamins, minerals and fibre. A good cereal supplies at least 5g of fibre per serving, which is usually 30g (1oz).

Focus on wholegrain cereals and those with bran or fortified with fibre. If you like muesli, choose low-fat versions, and compare the number of calories per serving, which reflects added sugars. Read labels and select cereals that contain the lowest amounts of sugar per serving.

BEST CHOICES				
Cereal	Portion	Calories	Grams of Fat	Grams of Fibre
Bran cereal with extra fibre	90g (3oz)	50	0.5	13.3
100 per cent bran	45g (1½oz)	80	0.5	8.0
Unsweetened shredded wheat	2 biscuits	160	0.5	5.0
Porridge	45g (1½oz)	163	3.3	3.6
Cornflakes	45g (1½oz)	173	0.5	1.5
Raisin bran	175g (6oz)	190	1.0	8.0
Wheat bran flakes with dried fruit and nuts	175g (6oz)	210	3.0	5.0

WORST CHOICES				
Cereal	Portion	Calories	Grams of Fat	Grams of Fibre
Sugar-coated cereal	115g (4oz)	120	2.0	0.0
Muesli (with nuts)	60g (2oz)	218	3.9	4.5

fibre per serving – about a third of the 25–35g a day experts recommend. Bran cereals, made from the outer layers of wheat, oats or other cereal grains, have the highest amounts of fibre. Overall, a daily diet high in fibre (from cereal bran, wholegrains, fruit, vegetables and pulses such as lentils) can help control your weight in several ways. For one thing, fibre itself has no calories. And since fibre is found only in foods from plant sources, high-fibre foods are often rich in nutrients and low in fat. Third, fibre-rich foods often take the place of higher-fat foods. And high-fibre foods are bulky, making meals more filling.

As a bonus, different types of fibre offer different health benefits. While the insoluble fibre in bran may help protect you from colon cancer, the soluble fibre in porridge may help

MAKE IT BETTER

Three-Grain Muesli

MAKES 4 SERVINGS

250 calories
•
1.5g of fat
•
(5 per cent of calories from fat)
•
3.5g of fibre

Despite its reputation for being healthy, muesli – especially the commercial variety – is often alarmingly high in fat and calories. Toasting the grains (which makes it more like the American granola and less like the European muesli) and adding honey help to make up for not using any added fat.

230g (8oz) puffed rice

175g (6oz) bran flakes

60g (2oz) porridge

30g (1oz) raisins

2 tablespoons toasted wheatgerm

120ml (4fl oz) unsweetened apple juice

2 tablespoons clear honey

Preheat the oven to 150°C/300°F/gas 2. In a medium bowl, combine the puffed rice, bran flakes, oats, raisins and wheatgerm. In a small bowl, stir together the apple juice and honey. Pour this over the puffed rice mixture and stir well. Use a non-stick tin 38 x 25.5cm (15 x 10in) or line with silicone paper. Spread the puffed rice mixture in the pan. Bake for 30 minutes or until golden brown, stirring twice during baking. Transfer the muesli to a large piece of aluminium foil. Let the mixture cool, then break it into pieces.

To store: transfer the muesli to a container. Cover loosely and store at room temperature until ready to serve. (Do not cover tightly because the cereal will not stay crisp.)

To serve: for each serving, place 90g (3oz) muesli in a cereal bowl and add 120ml (4 fl oz) skimmed milk.

Note: if you want to splurge a little, stir 30g (1oz) flaked or desiccated coconut into the cereal mixture before baking. You'll get an extra 35 calories and 2.4g of fat in each serving.

lower your cholesterol. To reap all the benefits of fibre, vary your choices of wholegrain cereal from day to day.

There's more: if they're fortified, breakfast cereals may supply a significant percentage of your RDA (recommended daily allowance) of some vitamins and minerals, including B vitamins (like folate) and iron. Some are calcium-fortified, helping you maintain strong bones underneath your nicely toned figure. Topping your cereal with milk or yogurt multiplies that benefit.

Here's how to make cereal part of a weight-smart breakfast.

Shopping Smart

Finding packaged cereals with the least fat and calories – and the most fibre – is easy: read the ingredients list and nutritional information on the packet. Pay attention to serving sizes: they vary from 1½oz (45g) to 3½oz (100g) or more.

Ready-to-eat cereal. Ready-to-eat cold cereal is a calorie bargain – provided you watch out for added sugars. To keep the number of calories down, don't get into the habit of adding a spoonful or two of sugar on your own.

Cooked cereal. Start with the best known – porridge (rolled) oats. Then look for other varieties, such as buckwheat, barley or a mixture of wholegrains. Try cooking dairy-free muesli like porridge. Quick-cooking and instant varieties save time – just add milk, heat and eat. Make them with water or skimmed milk for fewer calories.

Lean Menu-Makers

Cereal packets often list nutritional data for cereal with milk – for good reason. That's how we eat cereal. Stock your fridge and larder with other nutrient-rich ingredients that can be added with the milk.

- Fresh apples, peaches, pears, apricots, kiwifruit, bananas, berries – whatever fruit you like (to slice or spoon on top)
- Canned fruit in natural juices, not syrup (mandarin oranges, peaches, pears and apricots)
- Dried fruit (cranberries, cherries, apricots, apple slices, prunes and raisins)
- Chopped nuts (almonds, walnuts, hazelnuts) – use in small amounts
- Bran (to add extra fibre)

Eating Out

If you travel a lot, a steady diet of high-fat, high-calorie breakfasts can quickly add inches to your hips and waistline. Continental breakfasts may seem small, but croissants are full of fat even before you butter them. Cold cereal with milk and fruit is almost always on breakfast menus, even at fast-food places. If not, ask for it – it's often your best bet. When you're travelling, plan to eat a smart breakfast and have lunch, rather than wolfing down a late all-you-can-eat brunch. Chances are you'll eat fewer calories overall if you do this, because you won't be starving when you finally sit down for brunch.

CHEESE AND CHEESE DISHES

Cheese is apt to show up anywhere at mealtimes: in omelettes, sandwiches, soups, salads, casseroles, egg dishes, even in desserts or at breakfast. It varies in flavour and texture depending on many different factors: the milk used (from cows, goats or sheep), how the curds (or milk solids) are handled, whether it's aged (and if so, how), and whether any ingredients were added for flavouring. The results vary from plain old Cheddar to rich, tangy feta.

A compact form of milk, cheese has a similar nutritional makeup – plenty of protein and calcium, and a good supply of riboflavin (vitamin B₂). But a serving of cheese also contains more fat and cholesterol than a cup of milk. For most hard cheeses such as Cheddar or Edam, a serving is 1½oz (45g), about the size of six dice. That amount provides 300–400mg of calcium, 10 to 12g of protein and 12–14g of fat. A serving of processed cheese is 2oz (60g). This supplies about 350mg of calcium, 12g of protein (about 20 per cent of the RDA), and 18g of fat. Cottage cheese delivers calcium, too – about 75mg in a 2 oz (60g) serving; the fat content varies.

It's all too easy to nibble away at cheese, consuming more than we think. As a result, the calories and fat can add up. Reduced-fat versions of many popular types of cheese, including cream cheese, are available. If you prefer the flavour and cooking qualities of full-fat cheeses, eat small portions so that you can keep your fat and calorie intake within budget. Grate cheese, rather than using slices or chunks, to make a smaller amount go further. And make sure that most of your other food choices, including dairy foods, are lean, low in fat or fat-free.

Here are some other ways to go easy with cheese – and still enjoy its flavour and nutritional benefits.

Shopping Smart

Low-fat cheeses are good sources of calcium, so you get this bone-building mineral even while you save fat and calories. Whether you buy regular or reduced-fat cheese, check the nutritional information (if any), especially if you're salt-sensitive. The sodium content will vary. Also, cheese is perishable, so remember to check sell-by dates.

If you buy cheese from a specialist shop or at the deli counter, feel free to request nutrition information which must, by law, be available.

Here's how to select the low-fat cheeses that best meet your needs.

Cheddar, Swiss and other mature cheeses. You'll find reduced-fat versions of some, but not all, types of mature cheese. The melting qualities, texture and flavour differ from brand to brand. Some brands work better than others as substitutes for full-fat cheese. For pizza, lasagne and other Italian dishes, look for low-fat mozzarella.

Processed cheese. Cheese spreads and other pasteurised blends aren't ripened or matured. As a result, they don't have the same distinct flavour and texture. But they're versatile and keep longer than other cheeses.

Cottage cheese, ricotta and cream cheese. Often viewed as a diet food, cottage cheese may not be quite as low-calorie as many people think – even in this top item on most slimmers' shopping lists there are regular and low-fat kinds. Look for the one that's not more than 1–2 per cent fat. For salad dressings and dips, whip low-fat cottage cheese as a thickener or as a substitute for sour cream. Reduced-fat ricotta works well in baked dishes such as lasagne.

Also a soft, unripened cheese, cream cheese – the main ingredient in cheesecake – is very high in fat, so choose reduced-fat versions.

Don't count on cream cheese for calcium, though – it supplies very little.

Soya cheese. Made from soya protein, soya cheese (sometimes called tofu cheese) is a lower-fat, cholesterol-free alternative to dairy cheese. It doesn't taste much like cheese, however. Experiment to see if it appeals to you.

Lean Menu-Makers

If you find yourself turning to cheese as a way to put meatless meals on the table, be careful. Cheese is no lower in fat than meat – and may be higher. But with some careful planning, cheese dishes can be protein-rich main courses at brunch, lunch or dinner. Start with lower-fat versions of these

Best and Worst Cheeses

If you are trying to watch your fat intake, low-fat cheeses make excellent choices. Generally, cheeses that are lower in fat are also lower in calories.

BEST CHOICES			
Cheese	**Portion**	**Calories**	**Grams of Fat**
Grated Parmesan	2 teaspoons	20	1.5
Low-fat American-type processed cheese	1 slice	40	1.0
Low-fat Cheddar	30g (1oz)	50	1.5
Low-fat mozzarella	30g (1oz)	50	1.5
Low-fat cream cheese	30g (1oz)	56	4.7
Reduced-fat cheese spread	30g (1oz)	60	3.0
Low-fat ricotta	60g (2oz)	70	3.0
Low-fat (1–2 per cent) cottage cheese	115g (4oz)	90	1.5

WORST CHOICES			
Cheese	**Portion**	**Calories**	**Grams of Fat**
Mascarpone	30g (1oz)	124	13.0
Blue cheese	30g (1oz).	120	12.0
Cheddar	30g (1oz)	120	10.0
Cottage cheese (4 per cent)	115g (4oz)	120	5.0
Ricotta	60g (2oz)	110	8.0
Cream cheese	30g (1oz)	100	10.0
Brie	30g (1oz)	100	9.0
Cheese ball or log with nuts	30g (1oz)	100	4.0
Cheese spread	30g (1oz)	90	6.0
Feta	30g (1oz)	80	6.0
American-type processed cheese	1 slice	70	5.0

traditional cheese dishes, and pair them with a variety of the foods suggested here.

Macaroni cheese

- Mixed green salad (with fat-free dressing) and hearty multi-grain bread
- A salad of sliced tomato, fresh basil and low-fat mozzarella with a slice of crusty baguette

Toasted cheese sandwich on wholegrain bread

- Add sliced tomatoes to the sandwich and serve it with coleslaw tossed with fat-free dressing. For an interesting variation, try broccoli slaw
- A bowl of low-fat tomato soup and tabbouleh salad (a Middle Eastern grain salad) prepared with less oil
- Cucumber and courgette cut into sticks, and spring onions or chives

Cheese quiche

- Sautéed leeks or wilted spinach stirred into the quiche mixture before baking
- Steamed asparagus and a toasted slice of sourdough bread
- Stir-fried courgettes (if you keep them constantly on the move you need very little oil)

Weight-Friendly Substitutions

These low-fat kitchen tips can help you enjoy the flavour and texture of cheese without overdosing on fat and calories.

- In cheese spreads, extend a small amount of stronger-flavoured cheese, such as blue cheese, feta or mature Cheddar, with low-fat yogurt or cottage cheese.
- Substitute reduced-fat for full-fat cheese in your favourite recipes. Reduced-fat cheeses will melt better if you layer them between other foods or cover the dish while it's baking. Alternatively, you can use top-quality, full-flavoured cheese for half the amount of cheese in the recipe and a reduced-fat counterpart for the other half. This works particularly well with Cheddar.
- Use sliced soya cheese in sandwiches and lasagne and other baked dishes. Or grate it for casseroles and salad or soup toppings.
- Use soft tofu (a block of milky white soyabean curd) for cream cheese in dips, medium-soft tofu in cheesecakes, and sliced, firm tofu in sandwiches.
- Try light cream cheese or cottage cheese in cheesecakes.

Eating Out

When you order pizza ask for less cheese and more veggies. If you do treat yourself to pizza with pepperoni or sausage, limit yourself to just one or two slices: combined with cheese, high-fat toppings really add up.

Cheese sauces and toppings on baked spuds and other foods can add quite a lot of fat, too, especially if you're heavy with the ladle. Look for a fat-free alternative, such as salsa.

Many sandwich bars offer low-fat cheese if you're ordering in advance – just ask. Otherwise skip the cheese; order milk to get the calcium your body needs.

MAKE IT BETTER

Baked Macaroni Cheese

MAKES 4 SERVINGS

Per serving
•
415 calories
•
10.8g of fat
•
(24 per cent calories from fat)

This stripped-down version has 153 fewer calories and 24 fewer grams of fat than a standard version. For even more flavour, sprinkle a little grated low-fat Parmesan cheese on top and some fresh or dried herbs such as oregano. Use a reduced-fat Cheddar (or blend a strong-flavoured, full-fat mature Cheddar 50-50 with a reduced-fat one) and replace butter and whole milk with more reduced-fat cheese and skimmed milk.

230g (8oz) macaroni

1 tablespoon olive oil

1 tablespoon plain flour

½ teaspoon dry mustard

300ml (10fl oz) skimmed milk

150g (5½oz) low-fat mature Cheddar cheese, grated

115g (4oz) light ricotta cheese

2 tablespoons chopped spring onions

Salt

Ground black pepper

30g (1oz) toasted breadcrumbs

Preheat the oven to 190°C/375°F/gas 5. Use a non-stick 20 x 20cm (8 x 8in) baking tin. Cook the macaroni according to the package directions. Drain well. Meanwhile, heat the oil in a non-stick pan over low heat; stir in the flour and mustard. Cook and stir for 1 minute. Gradually stir in the milk. Bring to a boil; cook and stir for 1 minute. Add the Cheddar. Remove the pan from the heat. In a blender or food processor, purée the ricotta. Add to the sauce. Stir in the spring onions and pasta; add salt and pepper to taste. Spoon into the baking tin. Top with the breadcrumbs. Bake for 20 minutes, or until the top is golden brown.

CHICKEN, TURKEY AND GAME BIRDS

Sliced, diced, roast or barbecued, poultry takes the prize for versatility. By choosing the right cuts, using healthy cooking methods and being creative with herbs and spices, you can tempt your tastebuds, dodge fat and reap healthy dividends whenever you cook with chicken or turkey.

Poultry is loaded with protein, an essential nutrient that repairs tissue, bolsters immunity and helps keep your heart beating and your brain cells firing. While many other protein foods, such as beef and pork, can be high in fat, chicken and turkey shine because they're easily slimmed down by removing the skin, either before or after cooking. Three ounces (90g) of grilled or roast skinless chicken breast (a serving about the size of a pack of cards) gives you 53 per cent of your RDA for protein and just 3g of fat. It also supplies generous amounts of niacin (vitamin B), vitamin B_6 and iron.

Best and Worst Chicken and Turkey Selections

Unadorned, chicken and turkey are low in fat and calories. But how we order or prepare the two – fried, barbecued, roasted or souped up in dozens of ways – can drastically alter them (for better or worse). Here's a look at how some popular main courses measure up in calorie and fat content. (A healthy poultry main course should contain no more than 500 calories and 15g of fat or less.) The portions listed are typical servings for each dish.

BEST CHOICES

Main Course	Portion	Calories	Grams of Fat
Sliced, skinless roast turkey	90g (3oz)	133	2.7
Barbecued, skinless chicken breast	90g (3oz) with 2 tablespoons barbecue sauce	167	3.7
Grilled chicken kebabs	2 skewers	170	4.0
Roast, skinless chicken	1 leg and thigh, with buttermilk and breadcrumb coating	229	8.8
Grilled, skinless chicken breast	½ breast (90g/3oz), with rosemary and black olives	245	8.0
Chicken fajitas	2 fajitas with grilled chicken and peppers	318	5.0

WORST CHOICES

Main Course	Portion	Calories	Grams of Fat
Fried chicken (fast-food)	3 pieces (2 drumsticks and 1 thigh)	624	36.9
Chicken nuggets (fast-food)	12 pieces	573	34.6

MAKE IT BETTER

Spicy Roast Chicken Portions

MAKES 4 SERVINGS

Per serving
•
229 calories
•
8.8g of fat
•
(36 per cent of calories from fat)

This recipe contains 5.4 fewer grams of fat than the equivalent serving of a fried chicken thigh. To trim calories and fat from your other favourite chicken recipes, remove the skin and use egg whites instead of melted butter to make coatings stick.

120ml (4fl oz) buttermilk or low-fat yogurt

50g (1¾ oz) fresh breadcrumbs

1 teaspoon ground paprika

1 teaspoon ground black pepper

½ teaspoon dried thyme

1 small onion, finely chopped

4 pieces skinless chicken legs and thighs

Preheat the oven to 220°C/425°F/gas 7. Coat a wire oven rack with non-stick spray. Place the rack on a foil-lined baking sheet. Pour the buttermilk or yogurt into a shallow dish. Put the breadcrumbs in another shallow dish. Combine the paprika, pepper, thyme and onion in a bowl. Season the breadcrumbs with 1 teaspoon of the spice mixture. Add the remaining spices to the buttermilk. Coat the chicken pieces with the buttermilk, then roll them in the seasoned breadcrumbs. Place the chicken pieces on the prepared rack and coat them with non-stick spray. Roast for 15 minutes. Turn the chicken, coat it again with non-stick spray, and roast for 15 minutes more, or until golden brown.

Shopping Smart

Years ago, buying and cooking poultry was simple: you bought a whole bird, then either roast it or cut it up for other dishes. Today, you can buy various chicken portions, with or without skin, with or without bones, raw or precooked. Here's a look at how to make the best of what's available.

Boneless, skinless chicken breasts and thighs. Cut boneless breast meat into strips, then keep a package or two in your freezer. It will come in handy for stir-fries and pasta meals. Both breasts and thighs are good in most sauté recipes because they add very little (if any) fat to whatever sauce you have in the pan.

Chicken breasts, legs or thighs on the bone, with skin. These pieces are great for marinating and grilling because they hold in flavour and moisture. If you're going to baste the meat with a sauce such as barbecue sauce, remove the skin first to allow the sauce to cook in and flavour the meat more fully. Otherwise, remove it before eating.

Skinless chicken breasts or thighs on the bone. This type of chicken is best for roasting on a rack, as in the recipe on this page.

Whole chicken. Roasting chickens are meant for roasting, not frying or grilling. The whole bird generally has more fat than individual pieces without skin, so roast it on a rack to allow the fat to run off, and remove the skin before serving.

Turkey breast. Choose the real thing, not the processed version. (Processed turkey is a combination of pressed white and dark meat, and it's loaded with salt.) Roast it covered to lock in the moisture (turkey is a dry meat), and enjoy the leftovers in salads and sandwiches.

Turkey cutlets. If you can get these they are great lean sources of protein, perfect for grilling, sautéing and baking. Cutlets cook quickly and need some moisture, so marinate them, then baste with your favourite non-fat sauce – such as barbecue, teriyaki or sweet-and-sour – throughout cooking.

Minced turkey. Beware: regular minced turkey is no leaner than most minced beef, so reach for the extra-lean version. Three ounces (90g) of regular minced turkey contains more than 11g of fat, while the same amount of extra-lean light meat minced turkey has just 2.6g.

Lean Menu-Makers

Nearly every cuisine, from Italian to Chinese, uses poultry in some form. It's the most versatile meat around, simple to prepare in dozens of tasty ways. But don't let added ingredients and side dishes wipe out the healthy, low-fat benefits that chicken and turkey have to offer. Here are some of the best accompaniments for common cuts of poultry.

Boneless, skinless chicken breasts or turkey cutlets

- Pasta (linguine, penne, gemelli)
- Grilled or steamed Mediterranean vegetables (green or red peppers, mushrooms, aubergines, courgettes, shallots, green beans)
- Rice pilaf (brown, basmati)
- Oriental vegetables (mangetouts, water chestnuts, bean sprouts, pak choi)

Chicken or turkey breasts, legs and thighs on the bone, with skin

- Grilled onions and portobello mushrooms
- Steamed broccoli and cauliflower

- Steamed asparagus tips with lemon juice
- Glazed baby carrots
- Baked sweet potatoes
- Grilled pineapple slices

Whole bird

For roast chicken:
- Boiled new potatoes
- Carrots and parsnips
- Peas
- Mangetouts

For roast turkey:
- Steamed broccoli and carrots
- Baked squash
- Corn on the cob
- Brussels sprouts

Weight-Friendly Substitutions

Chicken and turkey are interchangeable in many recipes, and either one can often be used to stand in for other meats. Here are some suggestions.

- Enjoy extra-lean minced turkey in home-made burgers or chilli.
- Use turkey or chicken mince in place of minced lamb or beef for moussaka or shepherd's pie.

New Foods to Try

If you like chicken and turkey, try pheasant and quail. These are game birds and therefore low in fat; they are available at many supermarkets in season, or you can ask a butcher to order them. Although they cost more, these high-nutrition birds offer a unique taste sensation. Three skinless ounces (90g) – about the size of your palm – contains a skimpy 3.3g of fat and about 20g of protein. And there's no need to seek out exotic recipes for these birds: just roast them as you would a chicken or turkey. Or, for a low-fat, high-flavour treat, try pheasant cacciatore, prepared with mushrooms, onions and tomatoes and seasoned with herbs such as basil and oregano.

Two other members of the poultry family – duck and goose – are high in fat. Save them for special occasions.

Eating Out

When you're eating out, it often seems that the chef does everything possible to add fat to a dish. If you want chicken, ignore the menu and ask if you can have a boneless, skinless breast. If the dish comes with a sauce, ask for it to be served separately.

Salads with grilled chicken breast are a popular choice at many restaurants, but keep in mind that most dressings are loaded with fat. Substitute a reduced-fat dressing or ask for your salad to be served without. Alternatively, have it served separately so you can enjoy small amounts by dipping your fork in the dressing and then gathering a bite of salad.

CONDIMENTS, SPREADS, SAUCES AND JAMS

A stroll through any supermarket shows that we're a nation of condiment-lovers. Plain old ketchup, mustard and mayonnaise are just a start, leading into a kaleidoscope of marinades, sauces, spreads, relishes, sauces, dips, salsas and more. (see also Gravies and Sauces on page 58)

A typical dictionary definition of a condiment is 'a savoury, piquant, spicy or salty accompaniment to food.' Condiments and spreads concentrate flavour – and sometimes considerable fat and calories, if you're not careful.

If you're like most people, you probably rely a lot on condiments. You might use them to top your morning toast. Give a chicken sandwich oomph. Embellish a baked potato. Add character to salad vegetables. By the end of the day, you can accumulate a fair amount of fat and calories from condiments and spreads alone. Chosen wisely, however, they can add excitement and flavour for very little fat and few calories. Here's how.

Shopping Smart

If you've been trying to lose weight, you probably switched to fat-free or reduced-fat mayonnaise and 'diet' margarine years ago. And you probably already read food labels closely for fat and calorie counts. Here are a few category-specific tips to help make the most of the huge range of choices in the supermarket.

Reduced-fat mayonnaises. Good start: light brands contain only about one-third the fat of regular mayonnaise. The bad news is that both contain more fat than you want. So buy light, eat little, thin with skimmed milk to increase the volume, and for a flavour boost stir in some chopped garlic, onion or chives.

Butters, margarines and spreads. Butter and full-fat margarines are about as concentrated in fat and calories as a product can get. Just one tablespoon of either contains about 12 fat grams and 108 calories. As a table spread, 'calorie-reduced' or 'light' spread is your best bet, saving you 8.5g of fat and 73 calories per tablespoon over butter and full-fat margarine. Try different brands to find the flavour and texture that appeals most to you. Don't use reduced-fat spreads and margarines for cooking, though – they're high in water, so they won't brown foods, and they can ruin baked goods.

Look for margarine or margarine-like spreads made with olive or rapeseed oils. These products are higher in monounsaturated fats and are less likely to clog coronary arteries than other vegetable oils, which are higher in saturated fat, a factor associated with heart disease. Also, look for varieties that are free of trans fatty acids (by-products of the manufacturing process that make margarine solid at room temperature and affect your heart like saturated fats do).

Mustards. Go ahead – eat most mustards with wild abandon. Brown, yellow, smooth, coarse – most contain a scant 4–10 calories per teaspoon and virtually no fat. Be adventurous – try Dijon, Meaux and those with added herbs.

Best and Worst Condiments, Spreads, Sauces and Jams

As a general rule, try to limit the calories from condiments at any one meal to 50 or fewer. Be especially careful with jams (which weigh in at 40–50 calories or more per tablespoon) and peanut butter (at about 90 calories per tablespoon). If you use just a smidgen – no more than a couple of teaspoons of these spreads – you can enjoy toast, bagels and crackers without going overboard on fat and calories.

BEST CHOICES			
Condiment	Portion	Calories	Grams of Fat
Tabasco (hot pepper) sauce	1 teaspoon	1	0.0
Fresh lemon juice	1 tablespoon	4	0.0
Thick and chunky salsa	1 tablespoon	5	0.0
Prepared horseradish	1 tablespoon	6	0.0
Fat-free mayonnaise	1 tablespoon	10	0.0
Sugar-free jam	1 tablespoon	10	0.0
English mustard	1 tablespoon	12	0.0
Apple butter (see page 23)	1 tablespoon	15	0.0
Cocktail sauce	1 tablespoon	15	0.0
Ketchup	1 tablespoon	16	0.0
Sweet pickle relish	1 tablespoon	20	0.0
'Light' margarine-like spread	1 tablespoon	35	3.5

WORST CHOICES			
Condiment	Portion	Calories	Grams of Fat
Butter	1 tablespoon	108	12.2
Regular margarine	1 tablespoon	101	11.4
Full-fat mayonnaise	1 tablespoon	100	11.0
Honey mustard dressing	1 tablespoon	80	7.5
Horseradish sauce	1 tablespoon	60	4.5
Sandwich spread	1 tablespoon	55	5.2
Tartare sauce	1 tablespoon	50	5.0

For a sweet touch, try honey mustard, but be aware that one tablespoon contains 30 calories.

Tartare sauce, horseradish and relishes. Once you've switched to fish without butter, lean roast beef and low-fat sausages, you don't want to cancel out your calorie-saving efforts by smothering them in high-fat condiments. You won't go wrong here – provided you look for low-fat tartare sauce and prepared horseradish, not the cream variety. No luck? Just mix a handful of chopped herbs or some prepared horseradish with a tablespoon of light mayonnaise.

Jams and marmalade. Standard fare in most households, these are full of sugar – but not off-limits. Substituting one teaspoon of jam or marmalade for one teaspoon of butter or margarine on your breakfast toast cuts calories from your spread by more than half – from 36 to 16. The key is to buy the best strawberry preserve, orange marmalade, raspberry jam – whatever is your favourite – and then enjoy just a little. Or try low sugar (or sugar-free) jams or fruit butter (see page 23) for a lower-calorie alternative.

Bottled sauces. There are a huge number of flavour enhancers available for meat, chicken and fish: barbecue sauce, teriyaki, miso (a soya product), hoisin, soy sauce, Szechuan – plus the old favourites ketchup, brown sauce and Worcestershire sauce. Calorifically speaking, they're all pretty low – 4–8 calories per teaspoon – and they ring up a scant portion of a fat gram (compare that to Mornay sauce, at triple the calories and at least 2g of fat per teaspoon). Poured over lean beef, pork or poultry, these sauces will serve your weight-loss effort well, since they tenderise meat by breaking down animal protein.

Lean Menu-Makers

If you're like most women, meals at home probably centre around meat, pasta, potatoes, cooked vegetables and other basics. And you're probably short on time to prepare elaborate recipes. The right sauces and embellishments are quick ways to garnish mealtime standards without excess fat and calories.

Here are some quick and easy ideas for serving chicken, fish and vegetables.

- Pasta sauce with peppers, mushrooms and garlic
- Two tablespoons mustard mixed with one tablespoon balsamic vinegar (balsamic vinegar, incidentally, is an excellent low-calorie enhancement for plain grilled meat and fish and for salads)
- Two tablespoons of orange marmalade or apricot jam mixed with one tablespoon soy sauce
- One teaspoon peanut butter, one tablespoon soya sauce, and one teaspoon each chopped garlic and fresh ginger
- Fat-free mayonnaise and freshly chopped rosemary (one tablespoon each), and one clove garlic, minced
- Guiltless guacamole (two tablespoons mashed avocado; two tablespoons mashed frozen peas, defrosted; one tablespoon lemon juice; and chopped garlic, salt and pepper to taste)
- A roasted red pepper puréed with two tablespoons fat-free cream cheese and two tablespoons freshly torn basil
- Two tablespoons low-fat sour cream, one tablespoon lime juice, one tablespoon chopped fresh coriander and cayenne pepper to taste
- One fresh papaya, chopped, 2 tablespoons finely chopped red pepper, 2 tablespoons finely chopped green pepper, one teaspoon extra virgin olive oil and black pepper to taste

New Foods to Try

Consumers try ethnic dishes when they travel abroad. Food companies experiment with new varieties of condiments to suit our changing tastes. Growers respond by cultivating foods that are new to our diet but are widespread and healthy options in other lands. As a result, there are now more ways than ever to eat lean without ever getting bored or feeling that you're on a restricted diet. Consider trying some of these.

Margarine-like sprays. For most of these sprays, the main ingredient is soya bean oil. These brilliant inventions supply no calories or fat in the tiny amount needed to coat toast, a muffin or a serving of steamed veggies.

Soya margarines. Made from roasted soya beans, reduced-fat soya margarine contains about one-third the fat of peanut butter. When it's paired with their favourite jam even your kids will eat it.

Ethnic sauces. To lend an ethnic flair to standard meat dishes, try a Thai or Jamaican sauce. These are usually found on supermarket shelves near the soya sauce. You might be pleasantly surprised.

Salsas. The Mexican word for 'sauce', a salsa is traditionally based on a cooked or fresh mixture of tomatoes, peppers, onions and chillies. Fruit salsas make gentler accompaniments for chicken, fish and all sorts of vegetables. Start with mango salsa and grilled chicken – there will be no going back.

Hummus. A savoury combination of chickpeas and tahini, hummus is delicious spread on savoury biscuits or toasted pitta bread. Great if you're entertaining vegetarian friends (or avoiding dairy yourself).

Eating Out

More and more family restaurants are now offering fat-free condiments. You might also ask for a squeeze of lemon instead of butter- or cream-based condiments. This is a standard tactic – use it with no apologies.

If low-fat or fat-free alternatives are truly not available, you can minimise the damage by asking for your sauce or whatever to be served on the side. This tactic works well for Mornay, Hollandaise, tartare and other butter- or cream-based sauces, enabling you to take no more than you want.

Oriental sauces, on the other hand, are usually scant on calories, so they can be used fairly liberally – most have fewer than five calories per teaspoon.

DELI AND SANDWICH BAR FOOD

Office lunch hours often have to take in a haircut, collecting the dry cleaning or a supermarket dash, so a speedy sandwich is all there's time for. Be aware, though, that you can easily end up with a whole load of calories you don't want.

But it doesn't have to be that way. If the choices are vast – with lots of pasta and vegetable salads and reduced-fat meats – or if you can get a sandwich made to order, making wise selections is easy. Most of the time, however, you'll need smart-substitution skills to work out the best choices.

Shopping Smart

Here are some important things to keep in mind. The lowest-fat cold meats are turkey breast, chicken breast, roast beef and ham.

Sandwiches. If you like cheese, fine. But take in the guidelines on pages 31–4.

Be cautious when choosing an all-vegetable sandwich. Make sure those vegetables or salad ingredients aren't swimming in mayonnaise (in fact, always try to go mayonnaise-free if you can) or guacamole.

Finally, be savvy about the bread. Croissants make delectable sandwiches but are ridiculously high in fat and calories. Choose pitta, granary or wholemeal bread if possible.

Salads. Picking salads in the deli department is a real challenge. Chicken salad, egg salad, tuna salad, prawn salad – their common bond is mayonnaise. You're better off with lean meat as a sandwich filler. Or go for a mixed salad or try a bean salad.

Other Lunchtime Favourites. If you buy roast chicken pieces, remember to remove the skin because almost half the fat is found there. Drinks and desserts can easily pile on the calories. So take care with soft drinks, cappuccinos and fruity yogurts and choose spring water, black coffee or a piece of fruit instead.

Lean Menu-Makers

If you're in a supermarket you can easily buy vegetables and fruit for a healthy lunch.

- Bagged baby carrots, broccoli and cauliflower florets are good raw – an easy way to eat nutrient-rich vegetables at lunchtime.
- Buy an apple, banana or other seasonal fruit to round out your meal with no fat.

Best and Worst Deli and Lunchtime Sandwich Food

The first rule is: aim for plain. Choose unadorned meats, sandwiches and salads as opposed to those drowning in fat.

BEST CHOICES			
Food Item	Portion	Calories	Grams of Fat
Three-bean salad	115g (4oz)	78	2.4
Reduced-fat cheese	30g (1oz)	90	7.0
Sliced turkey	90g (3oz)	92	1.3
Sliced ham	90g (3oz)	93	3.0
Sliced roast beef	90g (3oz)	94	2.5
Roast chicken breast (without skin)	½ breast	142	3.1

WORST CHOICES			
Food Item	Portion	Calories	Grams of Fat
Fried chicken	¼ chicken	673	40.4
Crabmeat salad (in mayonnaise)	230g (8oz)	450	22.0
Chicken salad (in mayonnaise)	230g (8oz)	333	25.0
Potato salad (in mayonnaise)	230g (8oz)	325	17.2
Ham salad (in mayonnaise)	230g (8oz)	286	22.0
Pasta salad (in mayonnaise)	230g (8oz)	225	10.0
Salami	90g (3oz)	223	18.0
Corned beef	90g (3oz)	213	16.1
Egg salad (in mayonnaise)	115g (4oz)	209	16.0
Creamy coleslaw (in mayonnaise)	230g (8oz)	195	14.6

DESSERTS AND CAKES

Experts say that, for long-term weight control, you don't need even to try to give up desserts. You'll only feel deprived and go whole-hog when you do give in.

Chosen wisely, desserts can supply nutrients that you need. A pudding made with semi-skimmed or skimmed milk contributes calcium, for example. There are three rules. Make dessert calories count. Keep an eye on fat and sugar. And rein in the portions. Remember that 'low-fat' and 'fat-free' aren't a licence for second helpings. Eating twice as much can easily negate the benefit of choosing a low-fat version. Also, many reduced-fat treats more than make up for the calories from fat with added sugar. The fat-free versions may have even more calories than the regular versions.

Shopping Smart

To prepare low-calorie, low-fat desserts from scratch, stock the following staples. If time is short, buy convenience products. Where products state they are low-fat or fat-free, check the nutritional information on the package and compare the calorie and fat content to regular products. They may not necessarily have fewer calories.

Pantry staples. If you like to bake (or your family expects it), keep the following items on hand.

- Wholemeal flour, porridge oats and other wholegrains, such as barley flour to boost the fibre content in baked goods
- Low-fat dairy products for baked dishes
- Naturally sweetened fruit spreads and prune butter (see page 23) to replace part of the fat in baked goods
- Sugar substitutes. Read the tips for use on the package. Aspartame isn't appropriate for cooked or baked desserts

- Vegetable oil spray to coat baking pans unless yours are non-stick

Mixes. For quick homemade cakes and desserts, look for mixes with less fat or sugar (or, ideally, less of both).

Frozen desserts. Try lower-fat and fat-free varieties of ice cream as well as frozen yogurt, ices and sorbets, all of which are available in a variety of tempting flavours.

Packaged treats. Pop some low-fat, sugar-free biscuits in your shopping trolley. Read the label first to make sure they're really low-calorie.

Lean Menu-Makers

The following capture the essence of traditional puddings but with less fat and sugar than the originals.

Apple pie

- Baked apple (a cored cooking apple stuffed with porridge oats and brown sugar mixture and then baked)
- Apple flan (sliced apples topped with orange juice and slivered almonds and baked until just tender)
- Crisp apple and cheese slices (freshly sliced eating apples and reduced-fat Cheddar cheese)

Chocolate pudding

- Chocolate yogurt sundae (frozen chocolate yogurt topped with crushed low-fat ginger snaps)
- Chocolate smoothie (low-fat milk or low-fat frozen chocolate yogurt and a banana, whizzed in a blender until thick and smooth)

Weight-Friendly Substitutions

Try cutting back on high-fat and sugary ingredients. But take care: in many desserts, especially baked ones, substitutions affect the texture, volume and flavour of the end product. Experiment to get results that satisfy you. You may like your new version even better!

For baked desserts and cakes

■ Replace up to half of the fat with an equal amount of fruit purée, such as mashed banana or prune butter (see page 23). It imparts a naturally sweet taste, too, and adds to the moist texture. You can expect especially good results in loaf cakes and biscuits.

■ Use reduced-fat cream cheese in cheesecake.

■ Use fresh fruit or fruit canned in juice, rather than syrup, in fruit pies and crumbles.

Best and Worst Desserts and Cakes

Technically, you can have any dessert you like – provided you don't eat a large portion, eat it every day, or eat it several times a day. Also consider your food choices for the rest of the day. That said, if dessert appears frequently on your menu these guidelines will steer you towards choices that have less fat and fewer calories, especially when eaten in moderation. Select prepared desserts or choose recipes that have 25 per cent fewer calories per serving than the traditional versions. If you can find desserts that are also low-fat, that's even better.

BEST CHOICES			
Dessert	**Portion**	**Calories**	**Grams of Fat**
Poached fruit topped with toasted porridge oats	1 peach and 2 tablespoons porridge oats	55	0.0
Meringues	4 (about 20g/¾oz total)	73	0.0
Sorbet	115g (4oz)	80	0.0
Biscotti	1 biscuit (about 20g/¾oz)	100	3.0
Low-fat frozen yogurt	115g (4oz)	110	2.5
Brandy snaps	4 (about 30g/1oz total)	120	2.5
Strawberries with low-fat frozen yogurt	60g (2oz) sliced berries with 115g (4oz) frozen yogurt	122	2.5

WORST CHOICES			
Dessert	**Portion**	**Calories**	**Grams of Fat**
Cheesecake	1 slice (¹⁄₁₂ of 23cm/9in cake)	457	33.3
Fruit pie	1 slice (⅛ of 23cm/9in pie)	411	19.0
Tiramisù	115g (4oz)	390	23.0
Crème brûlée	115g (4oz)	362	27.2
Fruit crumble	115g (4oz)	360	18.4
Chocolate chip biscuits	4 biscuits	312	18.0
Premium ice cream	115g (4oz)	270	18.0
Iced cake	1 slice (⅛ of 20cm/8 in cake)	243	11.1
Fudge brownie	1 brownie (5cm/2 in square)	112	6.9

For toppings

- Instead of icing, top cakes with fresh sliced fruit, a spoonful of lemon yogurt or your favourite flavour of frozen yogurt.

- For a thick sauce, purée fruit with a little juice to the consistency you want. Try different types of fruits (mango, kiwifruit, blackberries or apricots) or a mixture. If you wish, thin the sauce with a splash of white wine.

- Dust cakes with icing sugar mixed with instant coffee, spices or cocoa.

For crusts

- Make pies and tarts with a single, not a double, crust. Or use a low-fat, prepared crumb crust.

- For a crumb crust instead of a pastry crust, coat the tin with vegetable oil spray, then dust it with low-fat digestive biscuit or amaretti crumbs.

- Before baking, top fruit with uncooked porridge oats instead of a pastry crust or crumble mixture.

For egg custard or milk pudding

- Prepare egg custard or rice pudding with low-fat milk and egg whites or egg substitute. Flavour with cinnamon and nutmeg or your choice of berries. Serve topped with sliced fresh fruit.

For any desserts

- Enhance the flavour with fresh or powdered ginger, grated citrus peel, mint or spices, and cut back on sugar, honey and other sweeteners.

- Substitute an equal quantity of low-fat plain yogurt in recipes that call for sour cream. (In fact, using the low-fat version of any dairy product helps cut calories.)

- For cakes and other baked chocolate desserts, replace melted chocolate with cocoa powder. Shave a little chocolate on top for flavour but few calories.

New Foods to Try

Dessert-lovers are notorious for trying new recipes. As you browse through your favourite recipe magazines, try recipes for these.

- Meringue shells flavoured with cocoa powder. Fill with low-fat vanilla yogurt and fresh berries or other fresh fruit.

- Soufflés made with egg whites and low-fat milk.

- Poached fruits flavoured with interesting spice blends.

As a ready-to-eat frozen dessert option, look in the supermarket freezer for fruit sorbet, frozen yogurt or a fruit water ice. Sorbet is easy to make at home, too, especially if you have an ice cream maker.

Eating Out

If you love to eat out and you love dessert, you may do better at upmarket restaurants than at fast-food places and family-style restaurants, where choices typically come with heavy whipped toppings, syrupy fruit fillings and thick gloopy icing.

Try these strategies for a sweet ending to your meal out.

- Fresh fruit: if it's not on the menu, you can ask whether they have any.

- Ask for sorbet (which has less fat, but is not necessarily low in calories) as a light, refreshing dessert – or a small, unadorned scoop of your favourite ice cream.

- Avoid temptation. A sneak peek at the menu or trolley makes it hard to resist. If you don't look, you're less likely to order.

- If you can't resist crème brûlée or tiramisù, order one dessert – with spoons for everyone at the table.

- For a little sweetness without too many calories, order coffee with either a splash of liqueur or crunchy biscotti or amaretti.

MAKE IT BETTER

Low-Fat Cheesecake

MAKES 12 SERVINGS

Per serving

•

121 calories

•

5.2g of fat

•

(37 per cent of calories from fat)

Light cream cheese, low-fat ricotta cheese and a crumb crust reduce the fat without reducing a forkful of flavour.

230g (8oz) light cream cheese

230g (8oz) low-fat ricotta cheese

2 eggs, separated

4 tablespoons clear honey

30g (1oz) sultanas

3 tablespoons cornflour

1 tablespoon grated orange zest

30g (1oz) amaretti crumbs

Preheat the oven to 200°C/400°F/gas 6. In a large bowl, combine the cream cheese and ricotta until smooth. Stir in the egg yolks, honey, sultanas, cornflour and orange zest, mixing until thoroughly combined. In a medium bowl, whip the egg whites with clean beaters for about 2 minutes, or until they form stiff peaks. Fold the whites into the cheese mixture. Coat a 22cm (9in) shallow pie dish with non-stick spray and press the amaretti crumbs on to it. Pour the cheese mixture into the pie dish. Bake for 30 minutes, or until golden and set. Serve cold.

EGGS AND EGG DISHES

Sitting unadorned in your refrigerator door, an egg contains about 5g of fat and 75 calories, including just 1.5g of saturated fat. Further, it offers a decent amount of protein – about 6g – plus riboflavin and other B vitamins, vitamin A, iron and other minerals. So it's a high-quality source of protein for vegetarians. In addition, eggs are an easy option when time is short, economical when you're on a tight budget, and flexible enough to combine with what you have in the fridge.

So far, so good. The problem, as many women know, is not fat or calories but cholesterol – a fatlike substance produced by the liver. All animals – including chickens – manufacture cholesterol. Your body does, too.

Although cholesterol contains no calories, a high intake of cholesterol in your diet is linked to high levels of cholesterol in your blood, which in turn is associated with heart disease. Experts advise limiting your intake of dietary cholesterol to 300mg a day.

Eggs contain more cholesterol than just about any food – 213mg in one large egg, all of it in the yolk. So it is best not to eat more than four whole eggs or egg yolks a week – that includes those in omelettes, quiches and so forth. Eggs are also used in baked goods and mayonnaise. (On the other hand, you can eat all the egg whites you want – they contain no cholesterol.)

You also want to keep a lid on high-fat,

high-calorie ingredients added during the preparation of egg dishes. Butter or margarine, mayonnaise, cream and cheese – all often found in egg dishes – can add significant amounts of fat and calories. And as it turns out, consuming a lot of saturated fat – the kind found primarily in butter and other foods of animal origin – contributes not only to your waistline but to blood cholesterol levels. But with careful planning, you can prepare egg-based meals while watching fat and calories.

Shopping Smart

Basically, you have two choices when buying eggs – whole eggs or egg substitute (you may have to go to a health food shop for the latter). Here's what to use and when.

Whole eggs. Eggs are sold as large medium, or small with corresponding differences in calories and nutrients. If in doubt for a recipe use medium.

Egg substitutes. These are blends of egg whites, skimmed milk, cornflour and vegetable oil, plus some vitamins and minerals. They look like raw beaten egg, and they contain no cholesterol and as little as 35 calories per 2fl oz (60ml). Check the nutritional information panel for calorie and nutrient content since some have fat, but others don't.

Use them to replace some or all of the whole eggs or egg yolks in your breakfast or in baked

Best and Worst Egg Selections

Eggs are a good source of protein and a medium size one averages 75 calories and 5g of fat – without added or accompanying fat. If you're watching your cholesterol intake as well as your figure, remember that a whole egg supplies 213mg of cholesterol. Experts advise consuming no more than four eggs or egg yolks a week. Keep in mind that many egg dishes can be made with low-fat or cholesterol-free ingredients.

BEST CHOICES			
Egg	Portion	Calories	Grams of Fat
Scrambled egg substitute	equivalent to 1 egg	35	0.0
Poached egg (yolk well-cooked)	1 egg	75	5.0
Hard-boiled egg	1 egg	78	5.3
Egg salad made with fat-free mayonnaise	115g (4oz)	98	5.3
Vegetable omelette made with egg substitute	substitute equivalent to 2 eggs	125	4.0

WORST CHOICES			
Egg	Portion	Calories	Grams of Fat
Cheese omelette made with full-fat cheese	1 serving (2 eggs)	356	32.6
Egg salad made with regular mayonnaise	115g (4oz)	190	16.3
Fried egg	1 egg	92	6.9
Hollandaise sauce	60ml (2oz)	86	8.0

MAKE IT BETTER

Basil and Mushroom Omelette

MAKES 1 SERVING

158 calories

•

6g of fat

•

(34 per cent of calories from fat)

Parmesan cheese and basil add a lot of flavour to this slimmed-down omelette. You could also make an omelette substituting egg whites for whole eggs and using other vegetables and herbs of your choice (such as broccoli and thyme). Use 2 real eggs if you cannot find egg substitute.

115g (4oz) sliced mushrooms

1–2 tablespoons fat-free stock

180ml (6fl oz) fat-free egg substitute

1 tablespoon water

½ teaspoon dried basil or 5–6 fresh leaves, torn

¼ teaspoon ground black pepper

1 teaspoon margarine

1 tablespoon grated Parmesan cheese

Gently cook the mushrooms in the stock, stirring frequently, until they soften and give up their natural juices. Then cook a few minutes longer to evaporate the liquid. In a medium bowl, whisk together the egg substitute, water, basil and pepper. In a medium non-stick frying pan over medium heat, melt the margarine. Swirl the pan to coat the bottom. Add the egg mixture. As the eggs begin to set, pull the outer edges towards the centre with a fork or spatula; allow uncooked mixture to run underneath. Continue until the eggs are just barely set. Scatter the mushrooms on top. Fold the omelette in half, sprinkle with Parmesan and transfer to a serving plate.

---

goods. Try several brands to find the ones you like, since the flavour and texture vary. Once the package is opened keep it refrigerated, and use within three days.

Egg replacers. For vegans, health food shops sell egg replacers, a mixture of potato starch, flour and leavening, which can substitute for whole eggs or egg whites. Just be aware that, without egg whites for consistency, dishes made with these products may lack the texture and flavour you expect from eggs.

Convenience foods prepared with eggs. Supermarkets sell partly and fully prepared products made with eggs: ready-cooked quiches pudding and cake mixes to name a few. These contribute protein and other nutrients you need. Check the nutritional information, and take cholesterol, fat and calories into account.

Lean Menu-Makers

Whether you use whole eggs, a combination of whole eggs and egg whites, or egg substitutes, don't let high-calorie accompaniments overshadow their benefits. Here are some serving suggestions for popular egg dishes.

Omelettes

- Fill with stir-fried vegetables, such as spinach, asparagus, peppers, onions, mushrooms and tomatoes, and serve with a granary roll.

- Fill with cooked, shredded chicken and serve with a tomato salad.

Scrambled eggs

- Top with chopped, fresh tomato and wrap in a wholemeal pitta.
- Serve on toast with a green salad.
- Stuff in a pitta pocket with shredded carrots and beansprouts, and serve with grapes.

Weight-Friendly Substitutions

The easiest way to work eggs into your menu without going overboard on calories or cholesterol is to prepare them without added fat.

For breakfast eggs

- Extend scrambled eggs by adding chopped, steamed vegetables just before the eggs are cooked, and use only one egg per person.
- To lighten scrambled eggs without adding fat, blend in a stiffly beaten egg white or low-fat cottage cheese.
- Cook scrambled eggs and omelettes in a non-stick pan that has been lightly coated with vegetable oil spray. That way, you won't need to add butter or margarine.

In other dishes

- Blend the eggs for egg salad with thick low-fat yogurt, cottage cheese or fat-free mayonnaise instead of full-fat mayonnaise. Add a touch of dry mustard, horseradish, paprika or snipped chives for flavour. Prepare the yolks of stuffed eggs the same way.
- To extend egg salad, mix in chopped celery or red or green peppers.
- Substitute chopped firm tofu for hard-boiled eggs for a mock egg salad.

- Replace whole eggs with egg whites or egg substitutes to cut cholesterol and save on fat. As a rule of thumb, two egg whites or 2fl oz (60ml) of egg substitute can replace one whole egg. This tip is as good for omelettes as it is for baked goods.
- For the colour and flavour of egg yolks, but less cholesterol and fat when a recipe calls for two eggs or more, use one whole egg and substitute two egg whites for the other egg.
- For totally egg-free baked goods, substitute half a small, ripe mashed banana or 1 oz (30g) puréed fruit for each egg called for in the recipe.

New Foods to Try

Using egg substitutes, try recipes for these dishes, all of which lend themselves to the use of substitutes.

- Huevos rancheros (Mexican scrambled eggs mixed with salsa and green onion, and topped with low-fat cheese)
- Egg drop soup (Chinese chicken broth, slightly thickened with eggs)
- Frittata (Italian omelette with the ingredients mixed into the eggs, not folded inside. It's finished under the grill, making it firmer)

Eating Out

If you regularly eat breakfast away from home, go easy on the cooked option. When ordering eggs, order one or two, rather than a three-egg omelette. To keep the total fat and calorie count down, have some fruit to fill you up.

Watch for other restaurant items made with significant amounts of whole eggs or egg yolks: baked custard, custard tart, crème brûlée, crêpes, flans, quiches and soufflés. Enjoy them – but share with a friend.

FAST FOOD

Believe it or not, you can still eat smart at fast-food restaurants (especially if they're not the mainstay of your diet). Among the standard greasy, salty, sugary fare are healthier options. See Deli and Sandwich Bar Food on page 41 for some extra ideas.

Shopping Smart

Look for nutrition information on the counter, on the wall or on the company's web site. If you have access to a computer, print out those pages and keep them in your car, so you can make your choice before you walk through the door.

Focus on bread, salad, fruit and milk. Pass up pastries, sugar and chips. For example, instead of fatty fries order a nutrient-dense mixed salad. A carton of milk would meet your dairy needs. Juice is better than a canned soft drink.

Burgers. 'Mega,' 'super' and 'jumbo' may give you a lot of food for your money. But you also get 'mega' fat and calories. A Big Mac has 560 calories and 31g of fat; a Whopper 660 calories and 40g. Instead, think in terms of reasonable portions – kid-size, if necessary. The regular hamburgers at McDonald's and Burger King have half the calories and a third of the fat of their overstuffed big brothers (and all, to be fair, supply iron, vitamin B$_{12}$ and zinc). Finally, pass up any special sauces.

Chicken and fish. These items aren't always a healthier choice than burgers. Pay attention to how they're cooked. Are they grilled without extra sauces and toppings? Or are they breaded or battered and fried? There's a huge difference in the amount of fat and calories. If chicken comes with the skin on, remove it. (At Kentucky Fried Chicken, for instance, a roast chicken breast without skin has 4g of fat; one with skin has 11). If good old fish and chips is tonight's takeaway supper, just strip off the coating and eat what is effectively healthy steamed fish. And go easy on the chips.

Baked potatoes. If they're available get a plain spud and top it with healthy salad-bar choices like onions, tomatoes and green peppers. Or order a small bowl of chilli to top your spud. At 7g of fat, it's a better choice than asking for the menu-item chilli and cheese baked potato (22g).

Salads and sandwiches. Lots of outlets now sell salads with fat-free dressings, and mayonnaise-free sandwiches.

Accompaniments. Ask whether low-fat versions of mayonnaise, salad dressing, milk and so on are available.

Indian and Chinese. Go for the simpler, less elaborate dishes (tandoori, for instance, and plain rice). And above all, don't eat too much – it's very easy to order lots of small dishes and end up with a feast for four.

Lean Menu-Makers

Milk. Round out any fast-food meal with a carton of calcium-rich skimmed milk, or ask for orange juice for a vitamin C boost. Either are better than a milkshake or fizzy soft drink.

Chips (French fries). Eat a small portion, or beg a few from a companion. Better still, go for a baked potato if you can.

Salad. Go for it! Use it to fill yourself up, but be careful with the dressing.

Fruit. Is there a bowl of apples behind the counter? (No, apple pie isn't a good alternative.) If there's really nothing on the premises, scout out fruit elsewhere for a healthy snack later.

Weight-Friendly Substitutions

Think small. You still may be getting too many calories and grams of fat for your liking, but at least the amount's not ridiculous. Small fries at

McDonald's, for example, tally 210 calories and 10g of fat – compared with super-size fries at 540 and 26. In general, choose plain and unadorned instead of 'supreme' or 'extra' or another qualifier that indicates a heavy helping of cheese, sour cream or special sauce.

New Fast-Food Options

Wraps. Wrap sandwiches are now popular and found everywhere. They are filled with grilled lean beef or chicken and lots of vegetables like tomatoes, peppers and onions. Don't forget beans – they're a nutritional goldmine.

Supermarkets. What could be faster than running in and grabbing a lunch-size pre-washed salad in a bag, a small piece of cheese, a packet of crispbread, and a couple of pieces of fresh fruit? Other good ideas: dried fruit, bite-size cereal, cereal bars and small cartons of milk or juice.

Best and Worst Fast Food

When your choices are limited, save fat and calories by choosing small portions of simple items.

BEST CHOICES

Fast Food	Portion	Calories	Grams of Fat
Burger made from minced lean beef (grilled, no bun)	90g (3oz)	166	6.1
Baked potato (with 60g/2oz broccoli and 2 pats of butter)	1 potato	244	8.5
Burger made from regular minced beef (grilled, no bun)	90g (3oz)	246	17.6
Small hamburger with bun (without condiments)	1 hamburger	260	9.0
Filled baguette with lean turkey, ham and vegetables (no mayo)	15cm (6 in)	280	5.0

WORST CHOICES

Fast Food	Portion	Calories	Grams of Fat
Nachos (with meat and cheese)	1 serving 310g (11oz)	770	39.0
Extra-large burger with bun, mayo, lettuce and tomato	1 burger	660	40.0
Extra-large French fries	1 serving	540	26.0
Cheese pastry	1 pastry	410	22.0
Grilled chicken sandwich (with mayonnaise)	1 sandwich	416	9.0
Fish and chips	1 serving	420	26.0
Pancakes and syrup	1 serving (3 pancakes)	440	9.0

FISH AND SEAFOOD

If you're a career dieter, you probably look first at the fish dishes on the menu when you eat out. And well you should: fish can be a helpful ally in your battle against fat. It's almost all protein, and because your body metabolises protein much more slowly than carbohydrates it keeps you satisfied for hours. The result? It helps you eat less over the long haul. Also, protein rebuilds muscle and powers the billions of chemical reactions that your body performs every millisecond, which is important in sustaining you during your body-shaping workouts.

Compared to other sources of protein, like meat or cheese, fish is relatively lean – from 2 to

Best and Worst Fish and Seafood

Fatty fish like salmon, tuna and swordfish have slightly more fat and calories than white fish like haddock and cod. But those calories are worthwhile – they supply omega-3 fatty acids, which are beneficial to heart health.

Whether you're cooking fish at home or ordering it when you are out, the key is to keep the added fat and calories from butter and cream sauces to a minimum, limiting the total number of calories from any fish dish to 150 and the number of grams of fat to 5. The exception: casseroles containing fish, where you need to allow for calories from all the other ingredients.

BEST CHOICES

Main Course	Portion	Calories	Grams of Fat
Steamed crabmeat	90g (3oz)	87	1.5
Haddock (grilled or baked)	90g (3oz)	95	0.8
Tuna canned in water	90g (3oz)	105	1.5
Steamed prawns with 2 tablespoons cocktail sauce	90g (3oz)	114	0.9
Tuna (fresh, grilled)	90g (3oz)	118	1.0
Grilled lobster tail with lemon juice	170g (6oz)	166	1.0

WORST CHOICES

Main Course	Portion	Calories	Grams of Fat
Fried clams with 2 tablespoons tartare sauce	170g (6oz)	600	42.4
Fried prawns	6–8 large	454	24.9
Steamed lobster tail with 2 tablespoons butter	170g (6oz)	370	24.0
Lobster salad	115g (4oz)	286	16.6
Battered fried fish	90g (3oz)	197	10.4
Canned tuna in oil	90g (3oz)	158	6.8

8 per cent fat, depending on the type, while a well-marbled porterhouse steak weighs in at 48 per cent fat. Trouble only arises when fish comes gift-wrapped in high-calorie coatings.

Shopping Smart

While fresh is the most delectable way to enjoy fish, there are plenty of convenient ways to include it in your diet. They now include low-fat options.

Canned fish. Water-packed tuna has 53 fewer calories and 5.3 fewer grams of fat than oil-packed tuna. Look also for water-packed versions of salmon and clams. If you like sardines and anchovies, save them for special occasions. They supply as many as 180 calories and 12g of fat for 3 oz (90g), even for sardines packed in tomato sauce.

As for tuna salad, if you make it at home with fat-free mayo you're in the clear. Tuna salads from the supermarket or sandwich bar, though, can be heavy on the regular mayonnaise.

Frozen fish. At one time, you simply couldn't get frozen fish without a calorie-rich bread coating unless you were happy to settle for prawns every time. It's still not universally available, but the bigger frozen food outlets stock it.

Throw a couple of fillets on the grill with some lemon and herbs, and you've added zero fat and calories but a whole lot of zip in just minutes. Or whip up a chowder-style thick fish soup with skimmed milk.

If you can afford them, buy prawns, lobster or crab. Although these crustaceans are higher in cholesterol than most fish, studies have shown that eating shrimps or prawns, for example, lowers triglyceride levels and raises high-density lipoprotein (HDL) cholesterol levels (the good variety). Ten large steamed or grilled prawns contain just 54 calories and barely a half gram of fat. If consumed without butter, even lobster – the Rolls-Royce of seafood – is totally figure-friendly.

Lean Menu-Makers

From salsas to cocktail sauce, there are plenty of fat-free and low-fat ways to spice up your fish fillet. If you're adventurous in the kitchen try making your own chunky salsa, stirring together chopped mango, orange or tangerine chunks, kiwifruit bits, chopped green onions and perhaps a dash of chilli powder.

- Fat-free salad dressings can double as interesting fish marinades. Experiment with your favourites. Give the fish at least an hour in the refrigerator to absorb the flavour, then grill.

- While most cocktail sauces are very low in fat, tartare sauces aren't – they're basically mayonnaise. If you're hankering for a good lower-fat tartare sauce, try making a simple version at home: add pickle to fat-free mayonnaise (to taste) and squeeze in some lemon juice.

- For a low-fat crabmeat salad, layer cos or iceberg lettuce with crabmeat and sandwich between two slices of wholemeal bread. Make the spread with low-fat mayonnaise, extending one tablespoon (an acceptable amount) with a little lemon or lime juice (and an artificial sweetener or dash of sugar as necessary). Fold in a grated carrot and chopped red onions.

- For an excellent low-fat meal in a bowl, see the recipe for seafood chowder on page 84.

Eating Out

Ever wonder why the grilled fish fillet from your favourite seafood restaurant is so moist? It's no secret: many restaurants add melted butter or herb-flavoured oils. To enjoy the lean benefits of fish, just ask for your fillet to be grilled plain. And take care with the accompanying sauces, which are usually high fat. If you must order them, ask for them on the side and eat sparingly.

For batter-fried fish, see Fast Food on page

50. You can compensate for the calories with exercise, but bear in mind that one indulgence demands nearly an hour of fast cycling.

Clam chowders and lobster bisques are made with cream, so if you must indulge share it with your dining companion. One cup of bisque, for example, comes in with nearly 200 calories and at least 8g of fat – that's about 25 minutes on the stairclimber at a fast pace. See page 84 for a good recipe for low-fat fish soup.

MAKE IT BETTER

Quick-and-Easy Tuna Casserole

MAKES 4 SERVINGS

Per serving
•
583 calories
•
12.8g of fat
•
(20 per cent of calories from fat)

This classic American recipe for low-fat comfort food can save the day on week nights when you haven't had time to shop but don't want to give in to fast food. Accompany it with grilled tomatoes – a great source of heart-healthy lycopene – or a salad of mixed lettuce, green peppers and beans.

230g (8oz) no-yolk or whole-wheat noodles

A 455g (16oz) package frozen broccoli florets, thawed

A 340g (12oz) can tuna in water, drained and flaked

A 300g (10³⁄₄oz) can fat-free, reduced-sodium condensed cream of mushroom soup

240ml (8fl oz) semi-skimmed milk

115g (4oz) low-fat Cheddar, grated

230g (8oz) low-fat plain yogurt

½ teaspoon ground black pepper

¼ teaspoon celery seeds

¼ teaspoon crushed red-pepper flakes

60g (2oz) reduced-fat snack biscuits, crushed

30g (1oz) grated Parmesan cheese

Preheat the oven to 180°C/350°F/gas 4. Coat a 32.5 x 23cm (13 x 9in) baking dish with non-stick spray. Cook the noodles in a large pot of boiling water according to the package directions. Drain and return to the pot. Remove from the heat; toss with the broccoli and tuna. In a large bowl, mix the soup, milk, Cheddar, yogurt, black pepper, celery seeds and red pepper flakes. Pour this over the noodle mixture and stir carefully. Transfer to the baking dish. Mix the biscuits and Parmesan; sprinkle over the casserole. Bake for 30 minutes or until lightly browned.

FRUIT AND FRUIT DISHES

If you love sweet things but your waistline can't afford to indulge frequently, fruit can help: it contains no fat and fewer calories than rich, sweet desserts. Keep a bowl of fruit handy, rather than chocolate, to snack on. Or drink calcium-fortified orange juice instead of cola.

To maximise the benefits of eating fruit, follow these tips.

Shopping Smart

A generation ago, most fruit was only available in season. While fruit is usually at its best then, you can now buy almost any fruit all year round.

Fresh fruit. Nothing beats a fresh, crisp apple or a juicy peach. Look for firm fruit, without bruises or signs of decay.

For a quick salad or snack you can usually buy cut-up fruit in the produce department of your local supermarket.

Canned or frozen fruit. For those days when you don't have time to shop, stock up on canned and frozen fruit like peaches, pears and pineapple. Canned tropical fruit salad is great stirred into low-fat or fat-free yogurt for an instant, delicious but nutritious pudding.

If the fruit is processed at its peak of perfection, the amount of nutrients may be greater than in fresh fruit that has been around

Best and Worst Fruit Selections

Try to eat two to four servings of fruit a day. 114g (4oz) of chopped fresh, frozen or canned fruit counts as a serving. So does 180ml (6fl oz) of fruit juice.

BEST CHOICES			
Fruit	**Portion**	**Calories**	**Grams of Fat**
Frozen unsweetened fruit	115g (4oz)	26	0.0
Canned fruit in juice	115g (4oz)	50	0.0
Mixed fruit	115g (4oz)	58	0.0
Fresh fruit, e.g. apple, pear	1 medium	60	0.0
Poached fruit	1 serving (half a peach or pear)	65	0.0
Fruit juice	180ml (6fl oz)	79	0.0

WORST CHOICES			
Fruit	**Portion**	**Calories**	**Grams of Fat**
Double-crust apple pie	1 piece (⅛ of a 23cm/9in pie)	411	19.4
Fast-food individual fruit pies	1 pie	266	14.4
Frozen sweetened fruit	115g (4oz)	100	0.0
Fruit-flavoured drink	180ml (6fl oz)	95	0.0
Canned fruit in heavy syrup	115g (4oz)	90	0.0

a while. Go for fruit canned in natural juices, which has fewer calories than fruit in syrup.

Dried fruit. Because moisture is removed, the natural sugars in dried fruit are concentrated. As a result, dried fruit contains more calories than an equal amount of fresh fruit. If you snack on them, you can quickly consume calories. Instead, toss smaller amounts of raisins, dried bananas, cranberries, prunes, apricots, figs, apples and so on into salads, breakfast cereals, pancake batters and mixed dishes (choose the no-soak kinds if you're going to eat them dry or uncooked – otherwise soak overnight in water, then stew until tender). Dried fruits are nutrient-packed, so by all means load some into your shopping trolley.

Fruit juice and fruit drinks. Check the nutritional information and ingredient lists for 100 per cent juice and juice blends. Fruit-flavoured drinks are mainly water and sweeteners.

Fruit bars, pastries and spreads. Fruit is an ingredient in all kinds of packaged and prepared foods – from dried fruit snack bars, to fruit spreads, jams and pie fillings. Many of these offer little in the way of fruit and much in the way of calories from added sugar, so opt for the real thing instead.

Lean Menu-Makers

Consider these imaginative ways to eat lean with fruit.

Fruit as the main event

- For breakfast, spread an array of sliced seasonal fruit or berries on a toasted English muffin and serve with hot chocolate.
- For lunch, serve mixed fruit in half a cantaloupe melon with low-fat or fat-free yogurt and raisin and hazelnut bread.
- Serve a bowl of chilled fruit soup (berry, melon, peach, mango) with a wholemeal roll and herbed low-fat soft cheese.
- For an elegant but light supper, fold mixed

fruit into a warm crêpe; top with plain yogurt.

Fruit as a mealtime supplement

- Add chopped fruit to main-dish salads – pears in chicken salad, apples in tuna salad and peaches in seafood salad.
- Add fruit to soup – grated, tart apples in lentil soup and orange juice and zest in carrot soup.
- Include dried fruit in grain dishes – dried cranberries in couscous and dried apricots in wild rice.
- Accompany main courses with fruit salsas – pineapple salsa with salmon, peach with chicken.
- Add fruit to vegetable salads – raspberries in spinach salad, chopped apples in broccoli slaw and tangerine segments in a mixed-greens salad.

Weight-Friendly Substitutions

What could be easier than substituting a fresh, crisp apple for apple pie? Fruit can be a menu item by itself – with no fat or sugar added. When you want something more, these quick tips can help you enjoy its nutritional benefits without sugar and fat.

As a sweet, refreshing beverage

- For no calories, replace sugary fruit drinks with ice-cold water flavoured with a slice of lemon, lime or orange.
- Enjoy plain juice instead of soft drinks for the nutritional benefits. Mix two juices together for your own refreshing blend.
- For a thick, creamy drink, blend fresh fruit with semi-skimmed milk or low-fat yogurt in place of ice cream. Half a banana, mashed, is a good thickener, too.

In fresh fruit salads

- Sweeten fruit with a few drops of vanilla extract or a light splash of juice rather than sugar. Combine mixed fruit compote with peach nectar or sliced pears with orange juice.

MAKE IT BETTER

Apple and Cranberry Crisp

MAKES 8 SERVINGS

Per serving
•
186 calories
•
5.2g of fat
•
(25 per cent of calories from fat)

Instead of viewing pudding as a sinful indulgence, consider it an opportunity to fulfil your daily fruit quota. This recipe for a healthy end to a meal focuses on fresh fruit, oats, wholemeal flour and apple juice concentrate, with minimal fat and sugar. If you can't get dried cranberries substitute other dried fruit, such as chopped prunes or apricots.

75g (2³/₄oz) porridge oats

40g (1¹/₂oz) wholemeal flour

60g (2oz) dark brown sugar + 1 tablespoon

Pinch of salt

Pinch of ground allspice

3 tablespoons chilled unsalted butter or margarine, cut into small pieces

3 large eating apples, cored and sliced into 6mm (¹/₄in) wedges

40g (1¹/₂oz) dried cranberries

3 tablespoons apple juice

Preheat the oven to 220°C/400°F/gas 7. In a medium bowl, combine the oats, flour, main quantity of sugar, salt and allspice. Using your fingers or a pastry blender, lightly mix in the butter or margarine until the mixture is crumbly. In a 20 or 23cm (8 x 9in) square baking dish, toss together the apples, cranberries, apple juice and remaining sugar until well mixed. Sprinkle the oat mixture evenly over the top. Cover with foil and bake for 20 minutes, or until the mixture is bubbly and the apples are tender. Uncover and bake for 5–10 minutes longer, or until the topping is lightly browned.

As a topping or sauce

- Purée fruit with a little juice to make a 'syrup' for pancakes. Try strawberries, peaches, blackberries and other less common fruits.

- Purée fruit with herbs or spices to make a delicious thick sauce for grilled chicken or seafood. For starters, blend mango with rosemary or peaches with cardamom.

To enhance flavour without adding calories

- Add grated orange, lemon or lime zest to soups, stews, salads and baked goods.

- In fruit dishes instead of sugar use spices that create the sensation of sweetness, such as cinnamon, ginger, nutmeg and cloves or a little vanilla extract. Some examples of spices that go very well with fruit are cinnamon on baked peaches, ginger in stewed apple, nutmeg in fruit soup and ground cloves in poached pears.

- Sweeten fruit and fruit dishes with sugar substitutes. However, aspartame loses its sweetness with heating and sugar substitutes may not give the result you expect in baked dishes.

New Foods to Try

Supermarkets now display a huge variety of fruit – you could go for a couple of weeks without eating the same fruit twice. Yet the average shopper sticks mostly with apples, bananas and oranges. When you can, try uncommon fruits such as mangoes, papaya, persimmons (sharon fruit), loquats, mangosteen, lychees or lingonberries.

To keep old standbys interesting, get creative: make up your own fruit salads and invent new smoothie combinations.

Eating Out

At restaurant buffets, choose fresh rather than stewed fruit, which is often prepared with plenty of sugar. When dining out means fast food, bring fruit with you. Skip fast-food fruit pies! At dinner, look for fruit options instead of a high-fat, high-calorie dessert.

When you're shopping, take a break and rest your feet while sipping a fruit smoothie, thickened with low-fat or fat-free yogurt or a banana, or a frozen fruit juice drink. Stick to regular sizes.

GRAVIES AND SAUCES

Good old-fashioned gravy made with meat dripping isn't such a hot idea – the calories and fat add up fast. But lighter versions are now available – and that goes for many other favourite sauces as well (see also Condiments, Spreads, Sauces and Jams on page 38).

Before you take that as licence to indulge, remember that many foods taste fine without embellishment. By preparing meat, poultry, fish and vegetables in ways that preserve their natural flavours, such as grilling or steaming, you do away with the need to tart them up. But for those times when something extra is called for, here are some tips.

Shopping Smart

Gravies. If you haven't looked at gravy mixes lately, you may be surprised at what's on offer. Flavours include pork, beef, chicken and roast vegetable. There are vegetarian options, with or without wheat, yeast, sugar and gluten. And some of them are fairly low-fat.

If the texture is too thick for your taste, thin the gravy with water, stock or wine when you heat it.

Creamy sauces. Let's face it: Béarnaise and hollandaise are diet-busters. If it's creaminess you're after, try reduced-fat condensed soups. Thinned-down cream of chicken, mushroom, celery and broccoli make good toppings for simply prepared chicken, fish and rice. Horseradish stirred into low-fat mayonnaise, yogurt or sour cream makes a superb sauce for roast beef. Replace the horseradish with dill for fish and seafood.

Other savoury sauces. Make leftover vegetables work for you. Purée cooked red peppers, broccoli or carrots with low-fat stock or wine. Start with ½lb (230g) vegetables and one tablespoon of liquid. Add more liquid if you want a thinner sauce or more vegetables if you want a thicker one, plus seasonings of your choice. This sauce can be used with meat, poultry or fish.

Tomato sauce (not ketchup) is good for more than just pasta. Chicken breasts, fish fillets and baked potatoes taste great with it. Look for those with least fat, or make your own by cooking skinned fresh tomatoes (canned if you prefer) with a very little olive oil and fresh or dried herbs of your choice, until the mixture has reduced and thickened. As for pesto, be careful. Even the reduced-fat type isn't what you'd call low in fat. The good thing about pesto is its assertive flavour – a little goes a long way. Thin it with low-fat stock or stir a spoonful into low-fat sour cream, yogurt or puréed cottage cheese. Then serve it with poultry, fish, steamed vegetables, baked potatoes or pasta.

Dessert sauces. Forget about custard and cream. Go for flavoured yogurt (add a little grated orange zest to enhance the flavour). Or try sweetening low-fat sour cream or plain yogurt with brown sugar. Don't overlook cranberry sauce, crushed pineapple, and puréed raspberries, strawberries, blackberries or other soft fruit.

Lean Menu-Makers

Naturally well-flavoured food requires little in the way of extra gravies and sauces. It pays to use the freshest, best-tasting ingredients you can buy and to prepare them in ways that preserve their flavours. For example, searing meat and fish over high heat at the beginning of cooking seals in juices and gives the surface an appealing brown colour. Little is needed to embellish foods cooked this way. Other flavour-enhancing techniques include: lightly steaming or microwaving vegetables until just crisp to conserve colour and taste – you won't miss the melted butter. Stir-fry vegetables with a splash of reduced-salt soy sauce. Pan-roast diced potatoes, courgettes, and aubergine with

Best and Worst Gravies and Sauces

If you're sizing up a sauce or gravy, those with fewer than 110 calories and 3g of fat are decent choices. Even meat gravy can make the grade – provided you don't empty the whole gravy boat over your plate. Dress it, don't drown it.

BEST CHOICES			
Gravy or Sauce	**Portion**	**Calories**	**Grams of Fat**
Tomato sauce	60ml (2fl oz)	18	0.2
Fat-free gravy	60ml (2fl oz)	20	0.0
Reduced-fat cream of mushroom soup	60ml (2fl oz)	35	1.5
Regular meat gravy	2 tablespoons	40	3.0
Fat-free chocolate sauce	2 tablespoons	110	0.0

WORST CHOICES			
Gravy or Sauce	**Portion**	**Calories**	**Grams of Fat**
Pesto	2 tablespoons	155	15.0
Curry sauce with coconut milk	80ml (3fl oz)	140	15.0
Hollandaise sauce	2 tablespoons	135	14.0
Béarnaise sauce	2 tablespoons	120	12.0
Custard	60ml (2fl oz)	114	5.6
Regular meat gravy	60ml (2fl oz)	80	6.0
Cheese sauce	2 tablespoons	60	4.4
Béchamel sauce	2 tablespoons	51	5.0

MAKE IT BETTER

Thigh-Friendly Mushroom Gravy

MAKES 8 SERVINGS

Per 115g
•
(4fl oz) serving
•
33.5 calories
•
0.1g of fat
•
(3 per cent of calories from fat)

If the men in your family insist on gravy with their Sunday roast, here's one that won't wreck your eating plan. This velvety stand-in for giblet gravy will save you 46 calories and 6g of fat.

60g (2oz) celery, sliced

60g (2oz) carrots, chopped

60g (2oz) onions, chopped

3 cloves garlic, chopped

Pinch of dried sage

Pinch of dried thyme

2 400-g (14-oz) cans fat-free, reduced-salt chicken consommé

10g (⅓oz) dried mushrooms, rehydrated following instructions on package

30g (1oz) plain flour

¼ teaspoon hot-pepper sauce

Place in a large non-stick pan the celery, carrots, onions, garlic, sage and thyme. Coat with cooking spray, cover and cook over medium heat, stirring occasionally, for 10 minutes. Add the consommé and mushrooms. Cover and simmer for 30 minutes. Using a slotted spoon, remove the mushrooms. Chop finely. Pour the gravy mixture into a blender, add the flour and blend. Return to the pan and add the hot-pepper sauce and mushrooms. Reheat to boiling point.

---

a little high-quality olive oil and balsamic vinegar to bring out bold flavours often hidden by high-fat toppings. Before grilling, gently rub the surface of meat with a mixture of dried herbs or spices to impart great flavour.

Weight-Friendly Substitutions

Turn your back on unwanted calories with these stand-ins.

- Instead of cream sauce, slowly whisk one tablespoon of flour into ½ pint (240ml) of cold low-fat milk until smooth, then stir over medium heat until the mixture comes to a boil. Continue to stir for a minute or two to get rid of the raw flour taste. Season with salt and pepper plus your choice of herbs, mustard, low-fat Parmesan or other cheese. For glossy, somewhat transparent sauces, substitute cornflour for the plain flour, but use half the quantity.

- Prepare your favourite packet sauce mixes with low-fat milk and half the butter or margarine.

- When making gravy, degrease the meat or poultry juices with a fat-separating jug before continuing with the recipe. Thicken the juices with cornflour or plain flour stirred to a smooth paste in a little cold water.

- Instead of adorning broccoli or cauliflower with cheese sauce, toss with lemon juice or balsamic vinegar.

New Foods to Try

Admittedly, old food habits die hard. You may think it impossible to cut back on gravy and savoury sauces, especially if you cook for someone who grew up eating these with his meals. But other things can take their place. Flavoured vinegars, such as tarragon and raspberry, add zest without fat. So do mustards such as honey, peppercorn and Dijon, which are brilliant with meat. If they're not 'sauce-like' enough for you, mix them with low-fat yogurt.

Eating Out

The gravy you get in a restaurant will not be low in calories or fat. Ask for yours to be served separately so you can take as much or as little as you want.

Additionally, it helps to brush up on your sauce vocabulary, so you know what you're getting. Here's a selection of sauces commonly offered in restaurants.

- Béarnaise. Tarragon-flavoured first cousin to hollandaise. This thick sauce gets its start with egg yolks, wine and butter. Use sparingly.
- Béchamel. Flour, cream and butter make up this one. Go easy.
- Bourguignonne. Mainly red wine with a bit of bacon. One of the lower-fat sauces.
- Curry. Contains coconut milk, which is high-fat. Proceed with caution.
- Hollandaise. Thick and creamy, with egg yolks and butter. Reserve for special occasions.
- Peanut. A staple of Thai cuisine, peanut sauce provides heart-healthy monounsaturated fat – just too much of it. Have only a smidgen.
- Velouté. This sauce is flavoured by meat, poultry, fish or vegetable stock instead of cream or milk. But it still has fat as its base, so have it only occasionally.

MEAT

If you've been eating poultry and fish every night in the name of slimming down, you can spread your wings now. Leaner cuts of meat abound these days.

Giving up meat can, in fact, be a woman's downfall. It supplies the nutrients busy women need to keep going. Three ounces (90g) of cooked meat provides about half your daily protein requirement, and about a quarter respectively of your zinc, niacin and iron requirements.

Balance, variety, and moderation are the cornerstones of a nutritious eating plan you can stick with in the long run. That includes modest portions of beef, pork, veal, lamb and ham. Most women need only about 6oz (170g) of meat, chicken or fish a day; 3oz (90g) of lean meat a few times a week will do you more good than harm.

Shopping Smart

Start by keeping high-fat meats out of your shopping trolley. If lean meat is on special offer at the supermarket, buy plenty, use just a small amount now and freeze the rest in 3oz (90g) portions.

Because the names of cuts of meat vary regionally, the information that follows is of a general nature. Always buy the leanest cuts you can find – for beef, that means avoiding marbled meat and looking for the highest percentage of lean meat when purchasing mince. Veal and lamb are fine as long as the cooking method doesn't add fat and calories. Be especially careful with cuts of lamb as it is naturally very high in fat. Despite its reputation ham is also lean, as long as the exterior fat has been trimmed off. Bacon? Streaky, no. Back, yes – as long as it's trimmed first.

Lean Menu-Makers

Treat meat as an equal partner, not as the centre-piece of your meals. Combine it with lots of grains and vegetables for satisfying, lower-calorie meals. Additionally, alter your meat preparation and cooking techniques to curb calories.

■ Always trim as much fat as possible from meat before cooking.

■ Grill or roast meat on a rack. Fat will drip off into the pan and won't be reabsorbed.

■ Use non-stick cookware and non-stick spray to minimise the need for added fat when sautéing or browning meat.

■ Another idea for sautéing or browning meat: use a small amount of fruit juice, wine or stock.

■ Brown minced beef as usual, breaking up the meat as it cooks. Transfer to a colander to drain well, then remove even more fat by rinsing with warm water. Pat the beef dry with paper towels before continuing with your recipe.

■ Fat undoubtedly makes meat more tender and succulent. So tenderise lower-fat cuts of meat by marinating them in acidic liquids such as juice (orange, lemon, grapefruit, white grape,

Best and Worst Meat Selections

When you're choosing meat, it's generally better to concentrate on fat rather than calorie content. For example, bacon doesn't contain a lot of calories, but most of those calories come from fat, not protein.

BEST CHOICES

Meat	Portion	Calories	Grams of Fat
Lean roast beef	3 slices 90g (3oz)	120	4.5
Back bacon, trimmed	3 rashers 90g (3oz)	129	5.8
Pork tenderloin	90g (3oz)	139	4.1
Lean stewing steak	90g (3oz)	176	8.6
Grilled pork loin chops	90g (3oz)	181	8.6
Lamb shish kebabs	90g (3oz)	190	7.5
Beef and broccoli stir-fry	115g (4oz)	346	3.9

WORST CHOICES

Meat	Portion	Calories	Grams of Fat
Barbecued ribs	170g (6oz)	674	51.6
Veal cutlet	115g (4oz)	322	19.0
Beef stroganoff	185g (6½oz)	300	13.5
Salami (made with beef and pork)	3 slices (90g/3oz)	214	16.5
Regular bacon	3 rashers (20g/⅔oz.)	109	9.4

Slimline Quick Beef Casserole

MAKES 4 SERVINGS

Per serving
•
335 calories
•
6.9g of fat
•
(18 per cent of calories from fat)

When it comes to beef, a little goes a long way towards helping you shape up, especially when it comes with tons of soul-satisfying potatoes and vegetables. This streamlined recipe is great for nights when your only alternative might be a takeaway burger and shake.

4 small red potatoes, each cut into 6 wedges

1 medium turnip, cut into chunks

1 medium parsnip, cut into chunks

4 pearl onions, chopped

3 medium carrots, cut into chunks

120ml (4fl oz) drained canned tomatoes

420ml (14fl oz) defatted reduced-salt beef consommé or stock

1 tablespoon red wine vinegar

2 cloves garlic, crushed

1 bay leaf

½ teaspoon dried thyme

½ teaspoon freshly ground black pepper

340g (12oz) lean, trimmed sirloin steak, cut into 1cm (½in) cubes

1 tablespoon plain flour

1 tablespoon olive oil

In a large, heavy pan combine the potatoes, turnip, parsnip, onions, carrots, tomatoes, stock, vinegar, half the garlic, the bay leaf, ¼ teaspoon of the thyme and ¼ teaspoon of the pepper. Break up the tomatoes with the edge of a spoon. Cover and bring to a boil over high heat. Reduce the heat to medium and simmer for 25 minutes, or until the vegetables are just tender. Meanwhile, toss the beef cubes with the remaining garlic and the remaining ¼ teaspoon each of the thyme and black pepper. Dredge the seasoned beef cubes with the flour. In a large, heavy frying pan, warm the oil over high heat until it's very hot but not smoking. Add the beef and sauté for 5 minutes, or until the beef is browned on the outside and medium-rare on the inside. Add the beef to the vegetables, reduce the heat to medium-low and simmer for 5 minutes, or until the vegetables are tender and the flavours blended. Remove the bay leaf before serving.

pineapple, tomato or vegetable), vinegar, wine or vinegar-based reduced-fat salad dressing. Or combine juice with stock for a less fruity marinade.

- Combine 3oz (90g) of lean beef or pork per serving with a generous amount of vegetables for a stir-fry. Cook the meat with minimum oil in a non-stick pan. Add the vegetables and stir-fry until crisp-tender. Serve with cooked rice.

- Skewer meat to make it go further. Shish kebab any combination of meat (3oz/90g per serving is plenty) and vegetables. Serve with boiled or steamed rice.

- Prepare your favourite stew with half the required meat, substituting diced potatoes and carrots.

Weight-Friendly Substitutions

Reduce the amount of meat you use by trying protein-rich substitutes.

- Use marinated firm tofu in traditional meat and vegetable stir-fries. Serve with rice.

- Substitute any of the following for 1oz (30g) of meat: one large egg, 1oz (30g) chicken or turkey, 1oz (30g) fish or seafood, 4oz (115g) cooked dried beans (or lentils or split peas), 2oz (60g) low-fat cottage cheese, 8oz (230g) low-fat yogurt or 1oz (30g) tofu, tempeh or textured vegetable protein.

- Use your slow cooker to make meat and vegetable meals. The long, slow cooking time tenderises lean cuts.

- Substitute rice for half the meat in stuffed peppers.

- Replace some of the minced beef in pasta sauces and meat pies with minced turkey breast.

New Foods to Try

Feeling adventurous? Consider game. Venison and rabbit are exceptionally lean and are becoming more widely available.

Soya products, such as tofu and tempeh, have gone mainstream and are good replacements for some of the meat in recipes. Try them in stir-fries, chilli and pasta sauces. The same goes for textured vegetable protein, which mimics minced or cubed meat in shape and protein content.

Eating Out

Whether it's fast food or fine dining, there's generally more meat in one serving than you need. Before you take a bite of your steak, cut it in half. Ask for a doggie bag (or take your own if it's not that kind of restaurant), and put half the meat in it before you start eating. You'll then avoid the temptation of finishing off food solely because it's sitting on your plate.

Far Eastern food is increasingly fashionable, so go Japanese and save. Select shabu-shabu, a simmered dish with meat; sukiyaki, which is stir-fried; and yakitori dishes, which are grilled. Add plenty of plain rice and clear soup to fill you up.

At Mexican restaurants, fajitas are a good choice because they combine vegetables with the meat. Skip the sour cream and guacamole that may accompany them.

MILK AND DAIRY

Milk in its various guises is more than a beverage. It's a snack (cheese or yogurt), a condiment (cream cheese or sour cream) and a dessert (ice cream). For women, milk and dairy foods supply hefty amounts of calcium, much needed for strong bones, plus decent amounts of muscle-building protein and essential vitamins B_{12} and riboflavin. After all, you may want to banish your belly, butt or thighs, but not at

the expense of the bones underneath. So in your quest for a beautiful body you want to include milk and dairy foods in your diet.

If you're not careful, however, they can serve up lots of fat and calories along with those valuable vitamins and minerals. And if you have trouble digesting lactose, the sugar naturally found in milk, you can end up with bloating, abdominal cramp, gas or diarrhoea. In this

Best and Worst Milk and Dairy Selections

From the examples shown here, it's easy to see how choosing the right milk and dairy foods can make a big difference in the amount of fat and calories you consume.

BEST CHOICES			
Food Item	Portion	Calories	Grams of Fat
Skimmed milk	240ml (8fl oz)	82	0.2
Low-fat buttermilk	240ml (8fl oz)	99	2.2
Semi-skimmed milk	240ml (8fl oz)	118	4.0
Unsweetened fat-free yogurt	230g (8oz)	137	0.4
Soya milk	240ml (8fl oz)	141	2.8
Low-fat chocolate milk	240ml (8fl oz)	158	2.5

WORST CHOICES			
Food Item	Portion	Calories	Grams of Fat
Greek yogurt	230g (8oz)	299	2.3
Sweetened yogurt	230g (8oz)	230	3.0
Premium ice cream	145g (5oz)	220	15.0
Non-dairy coffee creamer	2 tablespoons	88	5.6
Full fat milk	240ml (8fl oz)	163	9.1
Single cream	2 tablespoons	60	6.0
Double cream	2 tablespoons	134	14.3
Full-fat sour cream	2 tablespoons	60	5.0

chapter, you'll find out how to sidestep both problems. (For information on cheese, see page 31.)

Shopping Smart

If you're watching your weight, you're probably already buying skimmed milk. With 8.1g of fat and 150 calories per 8fl oz (240ml), whole milk gives you almost as many calories and fat as a handful of potato crisps.

Skimmed milk. With less than 0.5g of fat and only about 80 calories per 8fl oz (240ml), skimmed milk can help you shed the pounds that shave off inches effortlessly.

If you've avoided skimmed milk in the past because it tasted watery to you, look for protein-fortified products – the extra protein gives them the rich body of whole milk, with less fat and fewer calories. Or make the transition gradually, via semi-skimmed.

Coffee creamer. Don't let the non-dairy tag fool you – coffee creamers do contain fat. If you drink coffee on a regular basis, you're better off using milk.

Sour cream. At 2.5g of fat and 28 calories per tablespoon, sour cream isn't so bad provided that you limit how much you use. By substituting the lower-fat version, you can either use more or save calories.

Cream cheese. A tablespoon of regular cream cheese has 5g of fat and 51 calories. In comparison light, or low-fat, cream cheese supplies 2.5g of fat and 35 calories.

Try fruit- or herb-flavoured low-fat versions, if you can find them, or make your own easily at home.

Yogurt. Shopping for yogurt can be complicated. The choices are mind-boggling: full-fat, reduced-fat, non-fat. With fruit or fruit syrup, or plain. With sugar, with artificial sweetener or unsweetened. Along with those choices come a huge range of fat and calorie totals. Still, scouting out yogurt you like is worth the effort. For busy women, a container of yogurt makes an instant power-packed mini-meal or snack – a much healthier substitute for pastries or vending machine snacks. Further, many women find yogurt easier to digest than milk thanks to the active cultures responsible for fermenting milk into yogurt.

Frozen yogurt and ice cream. Saving up calories for a daily dessert helps you stay on the lean eating track. It takes only about 150 calories to satisfy this desire for pleasurable food – just the amount in appropriately chosen frozen yogurt or ice cream. Choosing well means ferreting out not only the best calorie bargain but also the rich flavour that still satisfies in a controlled portion.

As for premium ice cream, save it to accompany the occasional hot low-fat fruit pudding. Use only a small amount, like a rich sauce, and enjoy each mouthful slowly.

Lean Menu-Makers

If you don't care to drink milk 'straight', there are plenty of other ways to work it into your eating plan.

Breakfast smoothie. Whizz together in the blender one cup of skimmed milk, one cup of frozen fruit (strawberries or raspberries work well) and one banana. This drink also makes a refreshing between-meal power snack.

Hot chocolate. Stir a tablespoon of unsweetened cocoa powder (which supplies less than 1g of fat) and a packet of artificial sweetener into a cup of hot skimmed milk. Or use a packet of fat-free, reduced-calorie hot chocolate mix. As an alternative, add a teaspoon vanilla extract and some artificial sweetener to a cup of hot skimmed milk.

Digestion-Friendly Substitutions

Milk sugar, or lactose, is made up of two other sugars, glucose and galactose. The intestinal tract releases an enzyme, called lactase, to break up the milk sugar. When this works well, you don't even know it's happening. But if you don't produce enough lactase, however, you will suffer from abdominal gas and sometimes diarrhoea. Fortunately, there are alternatives.

- Ask in health food shops about lactase-treated milk.

- Try soya milk, which is naturally lactose-free. Soya milk's taste has improved dramatically over the years, although its texture is often rough. To get the most bone-building power from soya milk, choose a variety that has been fortified with calcium, vitamin D and vitamin B$_{12}$. Look also for low-fat versions.

  Other non-dairy milks are also available, made from oats or rice. They tend to taste better than soya, and oats are good for your heart.

- If you have been taking antibiotics, they may have upset the natural balance of bacteria in your intestinal tract. If so, try acidophilus milk or yogurt, which are fortified with *Lactobacillus acidophilus* bacteria.

- Buy calcium-fortified orange juice.

Eating Out

Don't feel self-conscious about ordering milk occasionally when you eat out – it will help you get your quota of calcium for the day. After all, children do it all the time. But remember, the calories will add up if you frequently order milk while dining out.

As for sour cream, cream cheese and yogurt, very few restaurants carry the lower-fat versions. So order carefully, and don't feel you have to eat everything that arrives.

Finally, putting cream in your coffee can break your fat budget pretty quickly, especially if you linger over a pot of coffee with a friend. Ask for a jug of skimmed milk instead.

PASTA, SAUCES AND TOPPINGS

Capellini, Farfalle and Rigatoni. A firm of Italian solicitors? No. They're types of pasta – just three of dozens. And they're a dieter's dream, despite unfair accusations of being fattening.

Pasta is filling, low in fat, packed with energy-producing complex carbohydrates and generally cholesterol-free. It's also a good source of B vitamins. You can't go wrong with all that nutrition for about 200 calories for a large serving. Where you *can go wrong* is topping your tagliatelle with fatty carbonara, pesto or meat sauces. And watch out for the fillings in stuffed pasta.

Shopping Smart

Happily, you don't have to give pasta the boot when cutting calories. Just keep these things in mind when shopping.

Pasta. With so many shapes and sizes available, you can have pasta every night for

Best and Worst Pasta, Sauces and Toppings

When you're planning a pasta meal, aim for about 300 calories per serving and 4g of fat or fewer (although you can afford a few more calories if the fat content is much lower).

BEST CHOICES			
Pasta or Topping	**Portion**	**Calories**	**Grams of Fat**
Parmesan cheese	1 tablespoon	23	1.5
Pasta primavera (with garlic and oil, not a cream-based sauce)	About 3 tablespoons sauce over 150g (6oz) pasta (uncooked weight)	107	4.0
Pasta with clam sauce (water, clams, oil and spices)	60ml (2fl oz) sauce over 150g (6oz) pasta (uncooked weight)	169	5.5
Pasta	150g (6oz) (uncooked weight)	197	1.0
Linguini with red clam sauce	120ml (4fl oz) sauce over 150g (6oz) pasta (uncooked weight)	257	2.0
Pasta with marinara sauce	120ml (4fl oz) sauce over 150g (6oz) pasta (uncooked weight)	268	2.6

WORST CHOICES			
Pasta or Topping	**Portion**	**Calories**	**Grams of Fat**
Spaghetti carbonara	120ml (4fl oz) sauce over 150g (6oz) pasta (uncooked weight)	378	11.5
Cheese tortellini	130g (4.5oz)	268	10.9
Pesto sauce	60ml (2fl oz)	157	13.1
Meat sauce	60ml (2fl oz)	68	2.0

weeks without ever repeating a meal.

But check labels carefully when buying fresh pasta, especially stuffed types like ravioli. Fresh often contains eggs and is generally higher in fat than dried; fillings are usually high in fat.

Sauce. Stick with low-fat meatless tomato sauces rather than fat-rich ones like pesto. Even reduced-fat pesto can have 4g of fat in just one tablespoon. Fat content can vary widely among tomato sauces, too, so check labels. Look for sauces with 4g or less of fat per 4fl oz (120ml) serving. Be especially vigilant when reading labels for creamy sauces. Often the serving size has been reduced to 2fl oz (60ml) – less than you might actually use. Best of all: make your own.

Cheese. What's pasta without cheese (besides much lower in fat)? If it's just not Italian without, make it a really well-flavoured type. Packaged grated Parmesan and pecorino are OK at a pinch – there are even some reduced-fat varieties. But freshly grated has far more flavour, so you can actually use less and still get the great taste. Buy a thin wedge of really good cheese (like Parmigiano Reggiano or pecorino Romano) and grate it at the table. Tightly wrapped, it will keep in the refrigerator or freezer for weeks, so you can always have some on hand.

Lean Menu-Makers

To make a calorie-conscious meal, start with about 3½oz (75g) of pasta (dry weight) per serving. Top with 4fl oz (120ml) of fat-free marinara sauce that you've mixed with 2oz (60g) of lean minced beef or diced cooked chicken (leftovers work well for this) and 4oz (115g) of sautéed onions and mushrooms. Add an interesting salad of frisée, rocket and radicchio with fat-free dressing – and there's dinner. Other ways to feast on pasta without piling on the pounds:

- Heat a can of drained minced clams in a saucepan with chopped garlic and fresh parsley. Reserve a little of the liquid to moisten the pasta, instead of oil.

- Mix heated marinara sauce with puréed low-fat cottage cheese or crumbled firm tofu. You'll get creaminess and a pleasing texture without a lot of calories.

- Stir puréed or chopped red peppers into tomato sauce for an extra helping of beta-carotene (an immunity-enhancing vitamin) with hardly any calories.

- Prepare a quick soup by mixing cooked pasta shells, diced cooked carrots and celery, leftover diced chicken and reduced-salt chicken stock. Serve with a large fruit salad for a balanced meal.

- For each diner, toss together cooked spaghetti (3½oz/75g uncooked weight), one teaspoon olive oil, 4oz (115g) of cooked chickpeas and one tablespoon grated Parmesan cheese.

- Purée cooked vegetables with enough stock to make a light sauce. Season with herbs and toss with cooked pasta. Top with a pinch of Parmesan.

- Serve 2oz (60g) per person pasta (uncooked weight) as a side dish. Toss with fresh or dried herbs and one teaspoon of melted butter or grated Parmesan.

Weight-Friendly Substitutions

Here's how to cut fat in some of your favourite pasta recipes.

- Replace minced beef in pasta sauces with minced turkey breast. You'll save about 65 calories per 3oz (75g) portion of meat.

- Let steamed mushrooms, onions and peppers stand in for some of the meat.

- Dilute reduced-fat pesto with chicken stock, and always use pesto sparingly since it will never be truly low-fat.

- Make macaroni cheese at home with skimmed milk and reduced-fat Cheddar cheese (see recipe on page 34). Add chopped cooked vegetables for extra fibre.

Beef and Spinach Lasagne

Per serving

•

595 calories

•

12.5g of fat

•

(19 per cent of calories from fat)

A typical slab of lasagne can easily contain 24g of fat. This slimmed-down version will please the whole family, and you can stick to your Eating Lean plan.

455g (1lb) reduced-fat ricotta cheese

A 255g (10oz) package frozen chopped spinach, thawed and squeezed dry

½ teaspoon ground black pepper

½ teaspoon ground nutmeg

455g (1lb) lean minced frying steak

1 teaspoon crushed red pepper flakes

Pinch of salt

A 750g (26oz) jar fat-free tomato–basil sauce

A 230g (8oz) box no-boil lasagne or 230g (8oz) regular lasagne, boiled following the packet instructions

5 leaves fresh sage, coarsely chopped

230g (8oz) low-fat mozzarella cheese, grated

1 plum tomato, thinly sliced

5 large leaves fresh basil

30g (1oz) pecorino cheese, grated

Preheat the oven to 190°C/375°F/gas 5. Coat a 20cm (9in) square baking dish with non-stick spray. In a medium bowl combine the ricotta, spinach, black pepper and nutmeg. Mix well. Place a large non-stick frying pan over medium heat until hot. Crumble the beef into the pan. Cook, stirring to break up the meat, for 4–6 minutes, or until the meat is no longer pink. Drain off any accumulated fat. Add the red pepper flakes and salt. Mix well. Spread a third of the sauce in the prepared baking dish. Place three or four lasagne sheets on the sauce so their edges don't overlap. Top with half the remaining tomato sauce and all the beef. Sprinkle with half the sage. Top with another layer of lasagne. Spread the ricotta mixture over it and sprinkle with half the mozzarella. Top with a third layer of lasagne and the remaining tomato sauce. Cover with the tomato, basil and the remaining sage. Sprinkle evenly with the pecorino and the remaining mozzarella. Cover tightly with foil and bake for 20–25 minutes, or until bubbling and heated through.

- Make pasta salads with lemon juice or balsamic vinegar and low-fat yogurt instead of mayonnaise. Add tuna canned in water and chopped vegetables for a meal in a dish.

New Foods to Try

Try wholewheat and spinach pastas, which contain up to three times the fibre of regular pasta. Fibre is a dieter's friend, since it keeps you full longer. All sorts of other colours and flavours are available, from squid ink to beetroot and garlic. The more tasty the pasta itself, the less sauce you need. And don't forget the non Italian types of noodles, like Japanese soba (made from buckwheat flour), udon (made from wheat or corn meal), somen and ramen (made from wheat), rice, mung beans and others.

Eating Out

Italian food is synonymous with large portions, and few pasta items on menus are low in fat. Your best bet is pasta topped with plain marinara or fresh tomato sauce. If that's not appealing, order a starter-size portion of another pasta dish and supplement it with a large green salad with fat-free dressing or a large bowl of minestrone soup.

Avoid cheese-filled pasta dishes , such as cannelloni, tortellini and ravioli, and spaghetti carbonara. Some sauces that look light actually have a lot of oil in them – if in doubt ask how they were prepared. Stick with dishes featuring lots of fresh vegetables, such as pasta primavera, as well as low-fat protein sources like fish, prawns and clams.

PIZZA AND TOPPINGS

Everyone likes pizza. But how does it fit into your plan to slim down – and stay that way? Quite nicely, thank you. Pizza is a nutritional powerhouse. The crust contains B vitamins and complex carbohydrates for energy. The tomato sauce supplies carbohydrates, vitamin C, lycopene (a natural substance that appears to protect against cancer) and little fat. The cheese provides protein as well as calcium to strengthen your bones. Topped off with vegetables, pizza provides fibre and vitamin A. For even more protein add lean meat or seafood.

Fat is pizza's pitfall. That doesn't rule it out of your eating plan, however. With a bit of know-how, you can curtail pizza's calories.

Shopping Smart

It pays to purchase healthy pizza ingredients so you can concoct a nutritious and satisfying meal at a moment's notice – and for a lot less than at a restaurant or takeaway. Here's what to buy.

Crust. Look for refrigerated and frozen pizza pizza crusts. Check labels to find the lowest in fat. Don't forget packet mixes; prepare them with less oil than is called for in the recipe.

Sauce. Look for sauces with 4g or less of fat per 4fl oz (120ml). Try different flavours to give your pizza extra sparkle.

Cheese. Buy reduced-fat cheeses and limit to 8oz (230g) per large pizza. Mozzarella is standard, but if there's a really tasty full-fat hard cheese you love, such as Cheddar, feta, or blue get them. Just use less – it's easy when the cheese is packed with flavour.

Other toppings. Favour veggies like onions, peppers, mushrooms and a few olives. Buy super-lean minced beef or turkey breast, better meat choices than pepperoni, sausage and salami. Brown the meat in a non-stick frying pan and drain it well before sprinkling it over the crust. Fat-trimmed back bacon and lean ham can replace regular bacon.

Frozen pizza. Steer clear of frozen deep-dish pizza; the fat is out of sight. Pick the frozen thin-crust varieties. Enhance their nutrition by adding steamed or stir-fried vegetables, lean minced beef or diced cooked chicken. (Leftovers are excellent pizza toppings.)

Lean Menu-Makers

Having nothing but a bought-in pizza for dinner is a lost opportunity. Limit yourself to two slices and a substantial salad with low-fat dressing. Or serve a side dish like steamed broccoli or baby carrots.

Leftover pizza is a portable feast. Have a piece of fruit with a slice of reduced-fat pizza and you have a healthy, light meal to eat on the run.

For an instant pizza, top a horizontally sliced baguette or piece of pitta bread with fat-free pizza sauce and 1oz (30g) of reduced-fat cheese. Heat under the grill or in the oven until the cheese melts. Eat with a salad or fruit.

Weight-Friendly Substitutions

- Sun-dried tomatoes can stand in for pepperoni. They have a similar look and intense flavour but are much lower in fat. (Drain them of as much oil as possible or buy dried ones to rehydrate in water.)
- Instead of sausage, try aubergines, broccoli, spinach, tomato slices, artichoke hearts or courgettes. Pair drained crushed pineapple or fresh pineapple pieces with lean ham, or have prawns or clams instead of meat.

Best and Worst Pizza and Toppings

Pizza can fit in nicely with your Eating Lean plan. Your best bets give you less than 300 calories and 12g of fat per slice, including the topping. On the other hand, if you're on a 1600-calorie-a-day menu plan and you treat yourself to a deep-dish individual pizza, that amounts to more than one-third of your calories for the day, even without a drink. So plan accordingly.

BEST CHOICES			
Pizza	**Portion**	**Calories**	**Grams of Fat**
Thin crust cheese pizza with peppers, mushrooms and onions (fast-food)	1 slice (⅛ of pie)	190	8.0
Homemade pizza (with low-fat prepared pizza shell, fat-free sauce, 220g (8oz) low-fat mozzarella cheese and 220g (8oz) steamed vegetables)	1 slice (⅙ of pie)	211	3.1
Thin crust cheese pizza (fast-food)	1 slice (⅛ of pie)	225	10.0
Thin crust cheese pizza with 30g (1oz) fat-trimmed back bacon	1 slice (⅛ of pie)	268	12.0

WORST CHOICES			
Pizza	**Portion**	**Calories**	**Grams of Fat**
Deep-dish cheese pizza	one 18cm (7in) individual pie	625	44.0
Deep-dish pepperoni pizza (frozen)	one 18cm (7in) individual pie	525	19.5
Stuffed-crust pizza with any meat topping (fast-food)	1 slice (⅛ of pie)	440	17.0

- Skip the cheese and pile on more vegetables to take up the slack. If it's calcium you're concerned about, have a glass of skimmed milk with your pizza.

New Foods to Try

Select wholewheat crust whenever possible. It adds fibre and a nutty flavour to your pizza. Low-fat tortillas and pitta rounds make great individual pizza crusts.

Eating Out

It's Friday night, and cooking is the last thing on your mind. Your family are clamouring for pizza. How can you refuse?

Limit yourself to two slices. You can always take the leftovers home. Order only half the cheese. To make the pizza more interesting and nutritious, request double the amount of tomato sauce and at least two vegetable toppings. To avoid eating too much pizza, always order a large mixed salad and a low-calorie beverage or water. Nibble on the salad before your pizza arrives.

If you just cannot resist a high-fat pizza, don't despair. Eat only a slice or two, then make up by curbing your calorie consumption and exercising more in the following days. No single meal or food makes or breaks weight-control efforts. It's what you eat in the long run that counts the most. Cutting out all high-fat favourites actually creates a destructive dietary backlash that leads to weight gain.

MAKE IT BETTER

Perfect Pizza for Waistline Watchers

MAKES 6 SERVINGS

Per serving
211 calories
•
3.1g of fat
•
(13 per cent of calories from fat)

When you want pizza in a hurry, use a ready-made supermarket pizza crust and load it up with veg sautéed in minimal fat. Compared to pizza with regular cheese and pepperoni, you'll save 190 calories and 17g of fat per slice.

60ml (2fl oz) low-fat spaghetti sauce

1 pizza crust

30g (2oz) courgettes, thinly sliced

30g (2oz) yellow squash or aubergine, thinly sliced

30g (2oz) red onion, thinly sliced

30g (2oz) shiitake or white mushrooms, thinly sliced

30g (2oz) broccoli florets

30g (2oz) red pepper, thinly sliced

115g (4oz) mozzarella cheese, grated

2 teaspoons Romano cheese

Preheat the oven to 200°C/400°F/gas 6. Spread the sauce on the pizza crust and set aside. Spray a non-stick frying pan with olive oil spray. Add all the vegetables and sauté over medium heat until tender-crisp. Arrange on the pizza crust; top with the mozzarella and Pecorino. Bake for 4–5 minutes or until hot and bubbling. Let stand 5 minutes before cutting.

POTATOES AND TOPPINGS

Pity potatoes. Although one of our favourite foods, they don't get the respect they deserve – from dieters or anyone else. (Why are lazy people called couch potatoes? No respect for the humble spud.) The truth is they are tasty, versatile, convenient and nutritious. But much like pasta, potatoes are often maligned because of the fattening company they keep and because in the past carbohydrates were demonised.

That's a shame, because potatoes are a nutritional bargain. For about 150 calories, a baked potato contributes complex carbohydrates and fibre, supplies more potassium than a medium banana, and provides about one-third of your daily vitamin C requirement. All that for zero fat and cholesterol.

It all boils down to this: in their simplest forms, potatoes are innocent of all the fattening charges levelled against them. As long as you don't eat them too often in their high-fat versions – au gratin or fried, for

Best and Worst Potatoes and Toppings

When deciding how to serve potatoes, aim for 180 calories or fewer per serving and fewer than 4g of fat, including the topping.

BEST CHOICES			
Potato	Portion	Calories	Grams of Fat
Boiled potatoes	170g (6oz)	113	0.1
Oven-baked sweet potato wedges	115g (4oz)	117	0.1
Mashed potatoes with skimmed milk	225g (8oz)	124	0.2
Medium plain baked potato	160g (5.5oz)	145	0.2
Boiled new potatoes, skin on, tossed with 1 teaspoon margarine or butter	170g (6oz)	149	4.1
Medium baked potato with 1 tablespoon low-fat sour cream	160g (5.5oz)	165	2.0

WORST CHOICES			
Potato	Portion	Calories	Grams of Fat
Large baked potato stuffed with chilli and cheese	200g (7oz)	482	22.0
Potatoes au gratin	115g (4oz)	323	18.6
Potato crisps	60g (2oz)	304	19.6
Large chips/fries (fast-food)	170g (6oz)	259	12.6
Mashed potatoes with butter and whole milk	225g (8oz)	223	8.9

example – potatoes can certainly be part of your successful slimming plan.

Shopping Smart

Whenever possible, use whole fresh raw potatoes. Here's what to look for.

Fresh potatoes. Choose only the best. That means looking for spuds that are clean, firm, smooth, and regular in shape. Pass up any with wrinkles, sprouts, cracks, soft dark areas or green spots. Ask about different varieties at your supermarket. Long whites are good all-purpose potatoes with a waxy texture. Round whites and reds are good for boiling. Store your potatoes in a cool, dark, well-ventilated place, where they'll last for several weeks. Don't keep them in the fridge, and don't store them near onions or they'll go bad faster.

Processed products. Instant mashed potato and other mixes are certainly convenient. If you prepare them without added butter or margarine, they're actually low in fat. Their main drawbacks are low fibre, high sodium and no vitamin C. Think of them as stand-ins for when you don't have time to prepare fresh potatoes. If you must have chips, make sure you buy low-fat ones for oven baking. Treat potato crisps – even the fat-free ones – as just that: treats. They don't count as a vegetable!

Lean Menu-Makers

Baked, boiled or mashed potatoes can be low-fat fillers, actually helping you to avoid overeating higher-calorie foods. They go with just about any type of meat, poultry and fish. Here are some super supper solutions.

- Serve roast chicken or turkey with low-fat mashed potatoes. Add one or two peeled garlic cloves to the pan when boiling the potatoes. Mash the garlic along with the potatoes. Replace butter or margarine with low-fat yogurt or skimmed milk. For even more flavour, boil the potatoes in fat-free chicken or beef stock.

- Make quick, homemade warm potato salad for a picnic. Microwave sliced potatoes until tender and toss with lemon juice or balsamic vinegar and chopped spring onions.

- Another picnic special: toss sliced or cubed cooked potatoes with fat-free mayonnaise and chopped hard-boiled eggs (use only the whites for zero cholesterol and less fat). Add diced vegetables such as onions, red and green peppers and celery.

- Make a meal out of a potato. Scoop the flesh out of one large baked spud, leaving the skin as a shell. Mix with 4oz (115g) low-fat cottage cheese, 4oz (115g) chopped steamed vegetables, and fresh or dried herbs. Spoon into the potato skin and sprinkle with one tablespoon of reduced-fat Cheddar cheese. Heat in an oven or microwave until the cheese melts.

- Slice potatoes and mix with peppers, onions, mushrooms and herbs; wrap in foil and pop in a hot oven for about 20 minutes. Adding 3oz (90g) cooked lean meat or poultry to the veg makes this a complete meal.

Weight-Friendly Substitutions

Here's how to pep up potatoes without blowing your calorie budget.

- Top baked potatoes with one tablespoon of reduced-fat sour cream instead of butter and save 80 calories and 8g of fat.

- Mix plain low-fat yogurt, chopped cucumber, chopped fresh or dried dill, salt and pepper for a terrific topper. Other ideas: soya sauce and sesame seeds; stir-fried mushrooms and onions; low-fat cottage cheese mixed with chives.

- When eating fast food opt for a medium baked potato with one tablespoon of low-fat sour cream instead of 20 chips – you save 35 calories and 5.5g of fat.

- Cube potatoes and toss with a little olive oil

and a sprig or two of rosemary. Roast at 200°C/400°F/gas 6 for about 20 minutes, or until tender.

- Make your own potato crisps. Slice into very thin rounds and blot on kitchen paper to remove excess liquid, and toss with a drizzle of rapeseed oil. Place in a single layer on a baking sheet and bake at 200°C/400°F/gas 6 until crispy, about 10 minutes.

- Crinkle-cut chips absorb less fat than straight, and both are better than cross-cut or spiral shapes.

New Foods to Try

Look for speciality varieties such as Pink Fir Apple. Or try sweet potatoes, which are becoming increasingly available in supermarkets and street fruit and veg markets. They provide comparable nutrition to regular potatoes, with a bonus: beta-carotene, a substance converted to vitamin A by the body and considered a powerful weapon in fighting off diseases like cancer.

Sweet potatoes should be firm, with bright, uniformly coloured skin. There are several types of sweet potato. You can cook them as you would potatoes but their sweetness makes them even more versatile – you can also use them in puddings or pies. Yams, which usually have a dark, bark-like skin, vary in flesh colour and are equally versatile in cooking. Store both sweet potatoes and yams unwrapped in a cool, dry, dark place for up to a week.

Eating Out

You already know that a baked potato is a smarter choice than fried or mashed. To jazz up a baked potato, choose sour cream not butter. It contains 30 calories and 3g of fat per tablespoon versus butter's 100 and 11. Naturally, the calorie advantage will evaporate if you use a heavy hand. Even better, calorie-wise, are veg-based sauces and lemon juice.

When adding any fat to spuds, avoid mixing it in with the potato pulp – its flavour disappears and you end up needing more. Mash the pulp first, then add a small amount of topping for flavour with less fat.

Ordering a potato can help you avoid choosing a hearty main course. You can pair a large baked potato with grilled trout and a green salad with low-fat dressing for a lean yet satisfying meal.

Avoid any menu item whose description combines the words 'loaded' and 'stuffed' in the same sentence as potato. A large spud with chilli and cheese has 482 calories and 22g of fat. As for potato skins, if you must indulge, share them with your companions.

When it comes to bought potato salad, just walk on by. Without a doubt, it's concocted with copious quantities of full-fat mayonnaise.

SALAD DRESSINGS

For many women, 'salad' conjures up an image of limp lettuce, tasteless tomatoes and a pallid sliver of cucumber that leaves you famished. It's low in calories, to be sure. But it's also low in flavour, so it may not satisfy your appetite. But with a little imagination salads of vegetables, fruit, grain products and other lean or low-fat ingredients can be wonderful. They contain little or no fat. And besides their nutrients they can supply fair amounts of fibre, which fills you up without adding calories.

When it comes to 'dressing up' a salad, though, you need to proceed carefully. In one study of women aged 19–50, salad dressings were their primary source of dietary fat.

Shopping Smart

When time is short, the quickest way to put your salad on a diet is to stock up on bottled reduced-fat or fat-free dressings. If you have a few minutes, make your own. To create salad magic at short notice, keep a range of vinegars, oils and seasonings as well as yogurt on hand. Either way, here's what to look for.

Prepared salad dressings. Nearly every supermarket has shelves full of low-fat and fat-free salad dressings. Because manufacturers use starches and stabilisers as fat replacers, these dressings aren't entirely calorie-free. And with so much variety, the amount of calories varies. Check out the nutritional information and experiment to find which ones you like best.

Vinegars. Vinegar has practically no calories and can be paired with any oil – in proportions you control – plus a number of herbs and flavourings. Start with the basics: cider vinegar, red wine vinegar and white vinegar. Try dark, sweet balsamic vinegar for a unique, strong flavour that is great on green salad.

Oils. All oils contain about 14g of fat and 125 calories per tablespoon. The difference is the amount of saturated fat, not total fat. Olive oil is high in monounsaturated fat, which can help lower your total cholesterol count. Don't assume that 'light' olive oil has fewer calories – it's simply lighter in flavour, not fat.

To get the most flavour from the least oil on salads, choose stronger-flavoured extra-virgin olive oil, sesame oil, nut oils or herb-infused oils.

Seasonings. To keep your tastebuds stimulated boost the flavour of homemade dressings with fresh herbs from shop or garden. Tarragon, oregano, basil, dill, chives and parsley are basics. Keep fresh garlic on hand, too.

Lean Menu-Makers

Switching to low-fat or fat-free dressing helps put a lid on calories. But with a few nutrient-dense add-ons you can also pump up the nutritional value of these standard salads. Choose whatever (wise) dressing you like for these potato and bean mixtures. Make your own or scour the supermarket shelves for low-fat versions of French, Italian, Caesar and so on.

Potato salad

- Combine cooked potatoes with cooked green beans and chopped red peppers.
- Combine cooked potatoes with lean ham and chopped green onions.

Three-bean salad

- Toss canned, drained beans (flageolet, pinto and cannellini) with chopped yellow peppers and halved cherry tomatoes.
- Toss canned, drained beans (black, kidney and chickpeas) with chopped onion, canned (drained) sweetcorn and chopped celery.
- Dip asparagus tips, rings of pepper and courgette sticks in low-fat blue cheese dressing.

Weight-Friendly Substitutions

Using a supermarket low-fat or fat-free dressing is one way to cut fat and calories. Using less oil and more vinegar in vinaigrette is another. Here are some other suggestions.

In place of high-fat dressings

- Fill a spray bottle with a full-flavoured oil to spritz your lettuce lightly.

- Skip the oil and dress your lettuce with balsamic vinegar. Or try a flavoured vinegar that you can buy or make yourself.

- Toss salads with a splash of sharp juice – orange, tangerine, lemon, lime, pineapple or tomato work well – and freshly ground pepper.

- For a creamy, homemade dressing for coleslaw or potato salad, use plain low-fat yogurt thinned with skimmed milk and add chopped fresh herbs, such as chives, tarragon or dill.

- Purée low-fat cottage cheese in a blender. Add semi-skimmed milk and flavour with fresh herbs, low-fat Parmesan cheese and freshly-ground pepper.

To dress up dressing

- Toss any dressing with chopped soft herbs (tarragon, parsley, basil, chervil, chives or garlic), curry, poppy or celery seed, or capers.

Best and Worst Salad Dressings

You can dress your salad without any fat by tossing it with lemon or pineapple juice or a dash of balsamic or flavoured vinegar. Or if it's something creamy you're craving, try one of the low-fat or fat-free bottled varieties. Look for salad dressings that have 3 grams of fat at most and no more than 40 calories per serving. The serving size listed on the label is often quite small, so measure the amount you put on your salad carefully.

BEST CHOICES

Salad Dressing	Portion	Calories	Grams of Fat
Balsamic vinegar	1 tablespoon	10	0.0
Fat-free mayonnaise	1 tablespoon	10	0.0
Low-fat mayonnaise	1 tablespoon	25	1.0
Fat-free vinaigrette	2 tablespoons	35	0.0
Low-fat blue cheese	2 tablespoons	40	1.5

WORST CHOICES

Salad Dressing	Portion	Calories	Grams of Fat
Blue cheese	2 tablespoons	170	17.0
Honey-Dijon	2 tablespoons	150	15.0
Thousand Island	2 tablespoons	140	12.0
Regular vinaigrette	2 tablespoons	120	12.0
Regular mayonnaise	1 tablespoon	100	11.0
Caesar dressing	2 tablespoons	100	9.0

- Add a few teaspoons of plain or fruit yogurt to herb vinegar for a creamy version of vinaigrette.
- Blend a strong mustard or horseradish or a little bit of chilli sauce into vinaigrette, thinned yogurt or thinned low-fat sour cream.

No-fat ways to dress a salad

- Grate a little orange, lime or lemon zest or some fresh ginger over salad greens and poultry or seafood salad.
- Toss in some distinctively flavoured salad greens such as watercress, endive, rocket, radicchio or frisée (available at supermarkets with extensive produce sections).
- For pasta or green salads, toss in chopped sun-dried tomatoes or chopped hot chilli peppers.
- Toss green salads with edible flowers (purchased in the fresh produce section, not at the florist).

Eating Out

Many women automatically order salad when they dine out, assuming it's bound to be lower in calories. If you opt for high-calorie add-ons, however, a salad main course can weigh in at more than 1000 calories. To keep a restaurant salad from turning into a surprise calorie-fest, remember these tips.

- Order salad dressing on the side. Then add just a small amount to the salad.
- Ask for a fat-free or lower-fat dressing. If one isn't available, ask for vinegar and oil served separately so you can mix your own.
- Enjoy a starter salad as your main Add low-fat soup and a roll.
- If you're helping yourself from a buffet, build your salad with lower-fat ingredients such as broccoli, pepper, sliced mushrooms, tomatoes and cucumber. You might not even miss the dressing if you omit it!

MAKE IT BETTER

Creamy Blue Cheese Dressing

MAKES 8 SERVINGS

Per 2 tablespoons
26 calories

•

1g of fat

•

(37 per cent of calories from fat)

A lot of women think blue cheese dressing is off-limits when they're trying to lose weight. Au contraire! Blue cheese is so packed with flavour that by pairing a small amount with fat-free cottage cheese you can save 144 calories and 16g of fat. To adapt other creamy dressings, substitute puréed, fat-free cottage cheese or yogurt for sour cream or other high-fat ingredients and flavour them with garlic and herbs.

230g (8oz) fat-free cottage cheese　　*2 tablespoons skimmed milk*

2 tablespoons crumbled blue cheese　　*1 clove garlic, crushed*

In a blender or food processor, blend or process all the ingredients on low speed for 20 seconds. (The blue cheese will still be chunky.) To store, cover tightly and refrigerate for up to 1 week.

SNACKS

It's every dieter's dream: snack and lose weight. Pure fantasy? Not necessarily. Munching chocolate all day won't bring you closer to your goals. But there's a lot more to snack on than this – and it's stuff your belly, butt, and thighs will thank you for.

Smart snacks offer valuable nutrients along with satisfaction and comfort – vitamins A and C, fibre and more. For example, you can increase your folate intake with nuts, calcium with frozen yogurt and fibre with fig bars. Make the right choices, and you can really nibble those excess pounds away.

Best and Worst Snacks

Approach snacks like meals – choose foods with the least fat and the most nutrition. Obviously, nutrient-dense, naturally fat-free vegetables and fruit are smart snacks any time. Otherwise, try to choose snacks with no more than 3g of fat in a 100-calorie serving.

BEST CHOICES			
Snack Food	Portion	Calories	Grams of Fat
Tomato juice	240ml (8fl oz)	20	0.0
Baby carrots with 1 tablespoon fat-free dip	5 carrots	45	0.0
Dry-popped popcorn	3 handfuls	90	0.0
Cereal bar	1 bar	92	3.0
Baked tortilla chips	13 chips (30g/1oz)	110	1.0
Baked potato crisps	11 crisps (30g/1oz)	110	1.5

WORST CHOICES			
Snack Food	Portion	Calories	Grams of Fat
Jumbo chocolate bar	1 bar (7oz/200g)	1000	60.0
Premium ice cream	4oz (11.5g)	220	15.0
Macadamia nuts	1oz (30g)	203	21.7
Regular potato crisps	15–16 crisps (30g/1oz)	150	10.0
Banana chips	10–12 chips (30g/1oz)	147	9.5
Jumbo chocolate chip cookie	1 cookie (about 8cm/3in)	140	7.0
Regular microwave popcorn	3 handfuls	120	9.0

—— MAKE IT BETTER ——————————————

Chewy Oatmeal Biscuits

MAKES 36 BISCUITS

Per biscuit
76 calories
•
1.7g of fat
•
(20 per cent of calories
from fat)

If your kids are clamouring for biscuits, you can indulge them (and yourself) without guilt.

170g/6oz plain flour

1 teaspoon ground cinnamon

¾ teaspoon baking powder

¼ teaspoon salt

60g/2oz margarine or unsalted butter,
at room temperature

60g/2oz caster sugar

50g/1¾oz light brown sugar

1 egg

80ml/3fl oz skimmed milk

1 tablespoon golden syrup

1 teaspoon vanilla extract

150g/6oz quick-cooking porridge oats

90g/3oz raisins

Preheat the oven to 190°C/375°F/gas 5. Coat two baking sheets with non-stick spray. In a medium bowl combine the flour, cinnamon, baking powder and salt and mix well. In a large bowl combine the margarine or butter and both sugars. Using an electric mixer, beat on medium speed until light and creamy. Add the egg and beat for 2–3 minutes, or until light and fluffy. Add the milk, golden syrup and vanilla. Beat until well mixed. Reduce the speed to low and gradually add the flour mixture, beating until just combined. Stir in the oats and raisins. Drop the dough by level tablespoons on to the baking sheets, leaving room for each biscuit to expand as it cooks. Bake for 8–10 minutes, or until lightly browned. Transfer to a wire rack to cool.

Shopping Smart

To find nutrient-dense snacks, read more than the information about fat and calories on the label. Look for fibre, calcium, iron and other vitamins and minerals.

Consider the 'crunch factor' when choosing snacks. Crunchy foods like baby carrots, apple slices, radishes, cucumbers and pickles take longer to eat than soft cakes, for instance. And they tend to be satisfying, so you may eat less of them.

Cereal bars. These are fortified with good quantities of vitamins and minerals and are usually low in fat, but watch out for the sugar content.

Nuts. They're filled with fibre, iron and all kinds of trace minerals and immunity-enhancing nutrients. Their biggest drawback, of course, is fat (even though it's heart-smart unsaturated fat). But if you eat just a handful you can reap their nutritional benefits. Remember that 1oz (30g) is considered a serving.

Popcorn. Dry-popped popcorn has only 30 calories and no fat in one handful. Eat a bag of microwave popcorn and you've put away 33g or more of fat – over half of what you should eat in one day. If you can't resist, look for light or low-fat types. Even then, take a good look at the label. The entire bag contains roughly three servings, so if you're downing it by yourself you could get as much as 330 calories and 15g of fat.

Crisps. Save half the calories and all the fat by eating fat-free potato crisps. (Regular crisps pack 150 calories and 10g of fat in a 1oz (30g), 15-crisp serving; fat-free crisps have 75 calories and no fat.) Low-fat tortilla chips have 90 calories and 1g of fat in a serving, compared with 142 calories and 7.4g of fat for regular.

Lean Menu-Makers

Here's how to improve the nutritional profile of some of your favourite snacks.

- Turn a biscuit into a nutrient-filled mini-meal by combining it with a glass of juice or a piece of fresh fruit.
- Stir a spoonful of crunchy, vitamin E-rich wheat germ into a carton of fat-free yogurt.
- Spruce up rice cakes with a thin layer of nut butter or fat-free apple butter (see page 23).
- Jazz up dry-popped popcorn with a splash of Tabasco sauce.

Weight-Friendly Substitutions

For those with a sweet tooth:
- Fresh fruit (see page 55).
- Dried fruit (see page 56).

Other smart swaps:
- Chestnuts instead of peanuts. Roast them in the oven. Five chestnuts have only 103 calories and 1g of fat.
- Dry-popped popcorn instead of microwave.

New Foods to Try

A snack can be defined any way you want. Think beyond chocolate, crisps and biscuits.

Soup. Choose canned and instant soups that are high in fibre, like minestrone, lentil and Tuscan bean. Pop into the microwave for an instant snack.

Cereal. It's not just breakfast food. And even when sugar-coated, it's much more nutrient-dense than cake. Eat bite-size cereal right out of the box. You can even find convenient snack-size bags of some cereal.

Office Snacks

Your good intentions needn't be left at home when you head to work. Just take along portable snacks like the following.

Desk drawer delights. Stock up on crispbread, rice cakes, low-fat biscuits, dried fruit, reduced-fat peanuts or cereal bars.

For the office fridge. Keep yogurt, baby carrots or cut-up vegetables, salad in a bag, skimmed milk, hummus and low-fat cream cheese spreads. (Travel tip: these snacks work well in the car; pack them in an insulated bag or cooler with ice packs.)

SOUPS

Hearty or delicate, piping hot or refreshingly chilled, chunky or smooth, creamy or clear, soup can serve as the prelude to a nutritious meal – or as its centrepiece. Take minestrone: chock-full of vegetables and pasta, minestrone (Italian for 'big soup') is a hearty main dish for a wintry day. In contrast, chilled gazpacho – based on tomatoes, peppers and cucumber – is a refreshing starter in peak-summer heat. Both are low in fat and a great way to work in the five servings of vegetables and fruit a day that we all need. And they're just some of the many low-fat, nutrient-rich soups you can put on your table.

Because soup is sipped, not chewed, it takes time to eat, which is a benefit for people who tend to overeat at mealtimes. Studies suggest that people who start their meals with soup eat less

Best and Worst Soups

Depending on their ingredients, soups can be the source of many nutrients. When selecting soups to buy or prepare, your best choices are low-fat versions with 3g of fat or fewer per serving.

BEST CHOICES			
Soup	Portion	Calories	Grams of Fat
Miso soup	240ml (8fl oz)	35	0.0
Gazpacho soup	240ml (8fl oz)	56	0.2
Vegetable soup	240ml (8fl oz)	90	2.0
Minestrone	240ml (8fl oz)	120	2.0
Bean soup, made without bacon	240ml (8fl oz)	130	0.5
Chicken soup, made with defatted stock	240ml (8fl oz)	160	3.0

WORST CHOICES			
Soup	Portion	Calories	Grams of Fat
Potato soup, made with cream	240ml (8fl oz)	220	14.0
New England clam chowder	240ml (8fl oz)	200	13.0
Chicken soup, made with regular stock	240ml (8fl oz)	175	6.0
Bean soup, made with bacon	240ml (8fl oz)	172	6.0
Cream of mushroom soup	240ml (8fl oz)	170	13.0
Borscht, topped with sour cream	240ml (8fl oz)	152	5.0
Bisque, made with cream	240ml (8fl oz)	120	5.0

Make it Better

Hearty Seafood Chowder

Makes 4 servings

*Per serving
252 calories*

•

4.1g of fat

•

*(15 per cent of calories
from fat)*

Thanks to defatted chicken stock and skimmed milk, this chowder supplies nearly 9 fewer grams of fat per serving than conventional chowder made with butter and cream.

1.2 litres (2 pints) defatted chicken stock

2 large potatoes, peeled and diced

1 large onion, diced

1 carrot, diced

1 stalk celery, diced

1 tablespoon chopped fresh parsley

1 bay leaf

½ teaspoon dried oregano

¼ teaspoon dried tarragon

¼ teaspoon ground black pepper

230g (8oz) cod, cut into 2.5cm (1in) pieces

A large can of clams in water

240ml (8fl oz) skimmed milk

Put into a 3.5 litre (6 pint) saucepan the stock, potatoes, onion, carrot, celery, parsley, bay leaf, oregano, tarragon and pepper. Bring to a boil, then cook over medium heat for 15 minutes or until the vegetables are softened. Remove and discard the bay leaf. Ladle about half of the vegetables and about 240ml (8fl oz) of the liquid into a blender. Blend until smooth. Return to the pan. Add the cod and simmer for 5 minutes, or until cooked through. Chop the clams finely and add to the pan. Stir in the milk and heat briefly. If the chowder does not have a sufficiently creamy texture for you, stir in some low-fat dried milk.

---

food and consume fewer calories than those who do not.

Soup is versatile – the ultimate mix-and-match food. Vegetable soup can be loaded with vitamins A and C, folate and potassium. Hearty soups made with rice, pasta or other grains – chicken with rice or beef noodle – contribute complex carbohydrates plus some fibre (if made with whole grains). Soups like chowder that are made with milk fortify your diet with calcium. And soup can be a great way to extend poultry, meat and fish, yet get the protein, iron and B vitamins you need for the day. Finally, bean

soups, such as split pea or lentil, are satisfying ways to add meatless dishes to your menu.

To build your soup repertoire, know the lingo. *Broth or stock* – tasty liquid strained from cooking vegetables, meat or poultry in water – is low in fat, especially when chilled and skimmed of fat. *Consommé* is simply concentrated broth. *Chowder* is a thick, chunky soup associated with the American East Coast, made with milk or cream, or thickened with a flour-butter mixture. *Bisque* is a rich, thick soup typically made with a base of seafood, vegetables, butter and cream. (But don't worry –

you can 'de-fat' chowder and other rich homemade soups or shop for low-fat varieties.)

Shopping Smart

If you're like most women, you probably rely on ready-made soups for fast meals. Think beyond old standbys like tomato. For versatility, you can combine two prepared soups or add extra ingredients.

To find soups with the least fat and calories, read the nutritional information. Clear soups are usually lower in fat and calories than creamy ones. You'll also find low-fat and fat-free versions of cream of mushroom, cream of celery and other higher-fat soups. Very often, the heartier the soup the more nutrients you get.

Whether you make from scratch or buy prepared, these health-smart tips can help you stock a soup-ready kitchen.

Canned and packet broth or stock. Stock your pantry with vegetable broth and fat-free beef and chicken broth – they serve as the base for all kinds of tasty homemade soups. If you're sodium-sensitive (or cooking for someone who is), buy stock with the lowest sodium (salt) content. Or make your own salt-free stock, then chill and skim off the fat. Low-fat stock cubes (meat or vegetable) can also be useful additions to your store cupboard. Again, look for ones that are low in salt.

Ready-to-eat soups or condensed soups. Ready-to-eat soups simply need to be heated. With condensed soup some of the water is removed, so you need to reconstitute them before heating. For more flavour and nutrients, use milk, broth, vegetable juice or water left over from cooking vegetables instead of plain water.

Dehydrated soups. Most are low in fat. To prepare, just add hot water or stock.

Soup Up Your Soup

With a little creativity and a few simple items from the supermarket, you can add homemade flavour and a nutritional boost to low-fat soups. Here's what to look for.

- Canned tomatoes, especially flavoured with Italian herbs. Add to corn chowder for a chunky texture
- Pre-cut veggies (frozen, canned or fresh, including stir-fry medleys) or cooked leftovers. Add to potato soup or other extra-chunky soups
- Canned beans. To reduce the sodium content, rinse the beans under running water before adding them to the soup. Mix them into vegetable noodle soup or into tomato for instant minestrone
- Firm tofu (smooth, creamy white soyabean curd sold in blocks). The firm variety keeps its shape when sliced. Add to chicken noodle or vegetable soup
- Canned crabmeat, clams or diced chicken. Add to celery soup
- Chinese noodles or small pasta shapes and couscous. These are especially good in turkey vegetable soup
- Brown rice or barley. Mix into reduced-fat cream of mushroom soup
- Sun-dried tomatoes or dried or canned mushrooms. Dried varieties have more flavour. Try them in onion or bean soup
- From your freezer: diced cooked skinless poultry, lean minced beef, seafood or leftover cooked meat. Add them to vegetable soup for a hearty main-dish soup

To enhance low-fat soups further, garnish them with these easy toppings.

- Chopped chives, coriander or parsley. These are colourful ways to spice up low-fat chowder
- A dollop of plain, low-fat yogurt. Add for some extra calcium on split pea or black bean soup
- A few shreds of Cheddar cheese or a sprinkle of Parmesan. Cheese gives body to minestrone.

Lean Menu-Makers

Paired with a salad or sandwich, soup rounds out a meal without rounding out your hips or waistline. Serve a cup of soup as a starter, or a fruit soup as dessert. (In Japan, soup is served for breakfast.) Consider these accompaniments for your favourite soups.

Chicken soup

- Pitta bread pocket stuffed with vegetables and tangerine segments on the side
- A pumpernickel bagel with fat-free cream cheese, and an apple
- Chilled fruit salad and matzo crackers
- Pear halves filled with fat-free cottage cheese, and rye crackers

Tomato soup

- Grilled chicken and spinach salad with low-fat dressing and breadsticks
- Toasted low-fat Cheddar sandwich and sticks of red or yellow peppers

Vegetable soup

- Turkey sandwich on pitta bread and fresh berries
- Small crusty wholewheat 'bread bowl' (made from a hollowed-out wholewheat roll), topped with low-fat Cheddar cheese

Weight-Friendly Substitutions

If you're trying to slim, you don't have to throw out your family's favourite recipes for creamy soups. You can lower the fat and boost the nutrients with these simple tricks.

Cream-based soup

- Replace the cream with a calcium-rich alternative such as skimmed milk fortified with low-fat dried milk.
- For cold fruit soups, blend in low-fat yogurt (plain or fruit).

Thick, hearty soups

- Add raw, starchy vegetables such as grated potatoes or parsnips. Simmer until thickened. In a hurry? Mix in potato flakes or leftover mashed potatoes instead. When the vegetables in your soup are thoroughly cooked, blend half, then stir the purée back into the soup. Or stir in a small can of tomato paste. Simmer vegetable, chicken or beef soup with rice, barley, oatmeal or pasta, or try adding cooked, mashed beans.

Eating Out

For lunch or a light dinner, a starter of soup plus a salad with bread may be all you need.

Before ordering in a restaurant ask about the ingredients. Soup prepared without cream, cream cheese, sour cream, egg yolks, cheese, butter or oil is usually lower in fat. And remember that clear soups are generally lower in fat than cream soups. If you must have a cream soup, order a cup instead of a bowl. And if you are in a self-service restaurant or cafeteria and helping yourself, take one ladle of soup, not two.

Chapter 6

Menu Magic

To jump-start your shape-up efforts, follow this one-week meal plan. Using the food selections nutritionists rate as best, plus the 'Make It Better' recipes, you'll eat well and love it.

Designed by registered dietitian and food and nutrition consultant, Kim Galeaz, this menu offers three tasty meals a day, plus snacks, for about 1600 calories and 44g (25 per cent of total calories from fat) or less per day. Obviously you will need to vary them within sensible guidelines,

according to the season, where you live, what you like and what's available.

'This meal plan supplies lots of flavour and variety (so you don't get bored) and fibre (so you feel satisfied and full, and don't overeat),' says Galeaz. 'It also keeps you fuelled all day long, to maintain energy as you exercise regularly to lose weight and tone up. There's even plenty of room for sweets and treats.'

Monday

Breakfast

75g (3oz) Three-Grain Muesli (see page 29) with 120ml (4fl oz) skimmed milk
240ml (8fl oz) fresh grapefruit juice
Snack
1 banana

Lunch

½ wholewheat pitta pocket stuffed with 30g (1oz) lean cold ham
1 apple
30g (1oz) low-fat mature Cheddar cheese
1 teaspoon light mayonnaise
115g (4oz) green and red pepper strips

Snack

1 Chewy Oatmeal Biscuit (see page 81)
240ml (8fl oz) skimmed milk

Dinner

90g (3oz) spaghetti topped with 2 tablespoons low-fat commercial pasta sauce
115g (4oz) steamed courgette and mangetout
1 soft breadstick

Snack

1 small pot low-fat white chocolate or raspberry yogurt

Tuesday

Breakfast

240ml (8fl oz) vanilla fortified soya milk mixed with 1 tablespoon instant drinking chocolate
2 crispbreads
1 tablespoon light cream cheese
Handful of seasonal berries

Snack

1 tangerine

Lunch

Grilled turkey breast with shredded lettuce and sliced tomato
230g (8oz) broccoli coleslaw mixed with 2 tablespoons low-fat dressing

Snack

1 fresh pear
A few plain peanuts

Dinner

1 bowl Hearty Seafood Chowder (see page 84)

90g (3oz) plaice fillet, grilled with lemon juice and oregano

75g (2½oz) bow-tie pasta

115g (4oz) fresh steamed asparagus spears

Snack

240ml (8fl oz) low-fat drinking chocolate

Wednesday

Breakfast

1 poached egg on toast

240ml (8fl oz) skimmed milk

Snack

240ml (8fl oz) vegetable juice

4 wholegrain crackers

Lunch

Sandwich made with 2 slices multigrain bread, 60g (2oz) reduced-fat Cheddar cheese, sliced tomato and 1 teaspoon spicy mustard

Tossed green salad made with fresh spinach leaves, cos lettuce and 1 tablespoon chopped walnuts, topped with a sprinkling of balsamic vinegar and a squeeze of fresh lemon

1 medium-size mango

Snack

60g (2oz) low-fat hummus with 1 mini pitta bread

Dinner

Beef stir-fry made with 90g (3oz) lean steak strips and 230g (8oz) Chinese stir-fry vegetables

175g (6oz) brown rice

Slice of honeydew melon

Snack

1 slice Low-Fat Cheesecake (see page 46)

Thursday

Breakfast

1 small pot lemon low-fat yogurt mixed with 1 tablespoon wheatgerm

115g (4oz) fresh strawberries, sliced

Snack

1 Waistline-Friendly American-Style Muffin (see page 24)

Lunch

One 90g (3oz) veggie burger on a seed roll with fresh spinach leaves and sliced tomato

12 baby carrots

240ml (8fl oz) skimmed milk

Snack

240ml (8fl oz) bean soup

4 wholegrain crackers

Dinner

1 portion Spicy Roast Chicken (see page 36)

1 serving mashed potatoes made with skimmed milk and no butter

115g (4oz) steamed fresh broccoli spears

1 wholemeal roll

Snack

Small bunch of grapes

Friday

Breakfast

2 slices wholemeal bread, toasted and topped with 1 tablespoon peanut butter

1 slice cantaloupe melon

Snack

240ml (8fl oz) low-fat drinking chocolate

Lunch

90g (3oz) water-packed tuna, drained, served over mixed fresh spinach leaves, rocket, and red-leaf lettuce, with 60g (2oz) sun-dried tomatoes

1 serving Creamy Blue Cheese Dressing (see page 79)
3 medium slices fresh pineapple

Snack

2 low-fat chocolate digestive biscuits
240ml (8fl oz) skimmed milk

Dinner

1 serving Perfect Pizza for Waistline Watchers (see page 73)
2 soft breadsticks dipped in 120ml (4fl oz) low-fat marinara sauce

Snack

1 small pot low-fat strawberry yogurt drizzled with 1 teaspoon chocolate syrup

Saturday

Breakfast

1 Basil and Mushroom Omelette (see page 48)
1 slice wholemeal toast
1 teaspoon light margarine
240ml (8fl oz) fresh orange juice

Snack

1 small pot low-fat raspberry yogurt

Lunch

90g (3oz) grilled prawn kebabs made with half a carrot and half a pepper
170g (6oz) aubergine and courgette slices, grilled
115g (4oz) couscous

Snack

240ml (8fl oz) skimmed milk
1 kiwifruit

Dinner

1 serving Baked Macaroni Cheese (see page 34)
170g (6oz) steamed cauliflower

Snack

Handful fresh raspberries
2 low-fat digestive biscuits

Sunday

Breakfast

1 sesame seed bagel, toasted and topped with 1 tablespoon apple butter (see page 23 for a recipe)
240ml (8fl oz) skimmed milk

Snack

Handful of fresh blueberries
20g (¾oz) Cheddar cheese

Lunch

1 serving Beef and Spinach Lasagne (see page 70)
Spinach leaves and cos lettuce with 4 cherry tomatoes and 2 tablespoons skimmed Italian dressing
1 slice bread rubbed with a clove of garlic, then lightly drizzled with olive oil

Snack

30g (1oz) dried cherries or other dried fruit

Dinner

90g (3oz) lean boneless pork loin, baked or grilled served with Thigh-Friendly Mushroom Gravy (see page 60)
1 baked potato, sprinkled with celery salt
115g (4oz) steamed fresh green beans
1 wholemeal roll

Snack

150ml (6fl oz) light cranberry juice cocktail

Chapter 7

The Best and Worst Cooking Techniques

Plain grilled chicken breast, steamed vegetables and boiled white rice. You could live on a steady diet of it. But would you want to?

All the austere low-fat cooking in the world won't put you any closer to your weight goal if the food lacks appeal.

Research shows that it's the very sparseness of diet plans that dooms them to failure. However, 'flavourful reduced-fat cooking techniques can help get you off the diet roller coaster for good,' says registered dietitian and nutrition consultant, Elizabeth Ward.

That's the message for 52-year-old Sarah. You met her earlier, in chapter 2. She's the mother of adult children who spares no high-fat ingredients in her cooking, despite the fact that she and her husband need to lose weight.

In Sarah's Kitchen

Sarah knows losing weight is imperative but finds it hard to change her cooking habits after all these years. She's typical of many women her age who've been losing, and gaining back, the same unwanted pounds for years.

A quick look around Sarah's kitchen tells the story of her battle of the bulge.

Pantry panic. Her cupboard shelves strain under the weight of packaged noodle, potato and rice dishes, which Sarah prepares with butter and full-fat milk. Cans of gravy and stuffing mixes pair up with the meat and potatoes she and her husband eat frequently. Creamy canned condensed soups are the basis

for easy weeknight casseroles. Bottled pasta sauces are loaded with cheese and oils.

White vegetable fat is on hand for making moist, flaky baked goods. You don't even want to hear about the big bottles of oil on the bottom shelf. And Sarah's baking ingredients include nuts and chocolate chips, which are just as easily eaten as snacks as they are added to recipes.

Freezer folly. Sarah fills her freezer with beef and pork, including fatty cuts and sausages. There's lots of high-fat mince for casseroles and meat sauces. Cheese and meat ravioli are quick fare. Sarah's nod to lower-fat dinners is breaded chicken and fish fillets.

Refrigerator reality check. The fridge contents don't bode much better for weight loss. There's full-fat milk and although non-dairy creamer is used for coffee, it's hardly fat-free. Hard cheeses (including Cheddar), cream cheese and sour cream help Sarah serve up the sauces, casseroles and baked goods she and her husband love. On the plus side, Sarah sometimes enjoys low-fat cottage cheese and fruit for lunch, so both are plentiful here.

There's no shortage of eggs in this kitchen, because fried eggs with bacon is her husband's favourite breakfast. Sarah also needs plenty of eggs to concoct sauces, puddings and cakes. She buys butter for sautéing veggies, flavouring rice, making sauces and baking.

Vegetables do overflow their rack. But all too often, Sarah doesn't get round to them until they're past their prime. So she sautés them in butter or oil to make them palatable – or blankets them with cheese sauce. Like many busy women, Sarah uses convenience vegetables such as ready-sliced carrots and washed-and-bagged salad greens. Ideally, they're a smart way to boost vegetable consumption. But if you smother them with full-fat salad dressing as Sarah does, you cancel out their low-fat, low-calorie benefits.

Countertop confusion. On Sarah's countertop is a well-used deep-fat fryer. But frying is folly when weight control is the goal.

Cooking Light Lessons

Believe it or not, Sarah isn't a lost cause. In spite of her kitchen's fat traps, she needn't totally revamp her diet. Some artful substitutions of ingredients and cooking methods will go a long way towards getting her on track. Consider this: eating 100 fewer calories a day can result in more than 10lb (4.5 kg) lost in a year's time, provided you don't decrease your activity level. What does that mean in tabletop terms? Something as painless as cutting one tablespoon of butter or margarine from your daily diet. (Just use a little less on your toast or baked potato – you won't miss it!)

Baking

So many different kinds of foods can be baked that this cooking method offers the greatest opportunity for calorie cutting.

Main-dish misery. They're convenient. They're comfort foods. They're calorific killers. Main-course ovenbakes prepared with the traditional meat, cream, cheese and butter can bust your calorie budget. The good news? There are dozens of ways to lighten up such family favourites.

• For meat and poultry dishes such as shepherd's pie or moussaka, use no more than 90g (3oz) of meat per serving and remove visible fat before cooking. When browning mince, drain

off the fat that collects in the frying pan. Then get rid of even more fat by transferring the meat to a colander and rinsing it with warm water or blotting with kitchen paper. Better yet, start with lean minced beef or substitute minced turkey or chicken breast. Finally, replace some of the meat with cooked rice, couscous or beans, or with low-fat cottage cheese.

• Lighten up comfort foods like chicken fricassee and macaroni cheese with low-fat versions of milk, sour cream or yogurt. For baked pasta dishes use reduced-fat mozzarella, Cheddar, ricotta or other cheese. Aubergines absorb a lot of oil, so bake the slices instead of frying them before assembling any dish that contains them.

• Where recipes call for feta cheese substitute half with non-fat cottage cheese. Make your own non-fat substitute for sour cream by puréeing one cup of fat-free cottage cheese with one tablespoon of lemon juice in a food processor until perfectly smooth.

• Lighten quiche and soufflés by replacing some or all of the eggs with fat-free egg substitute or egg whites (use 2fl oz/60ml egg substitute or two whites for every whole egg).

• Prepare low-calorie sauces for creamy type casseroles by thickening fat-free stock or skimmed milk with cornflour or arrowroot. Or use low-fat versions of condensed soups like cream of chicken, mushroom, celery or broccoli.

Sumptuous fish and seafood. Baking is best for lower-fat fish, such as cod, haddock, halibut, plaice and sole. But be quick about it: lean fish loses moisture faster than its fattier cousins like salmon, herring and mackerel. One good no-fat technique is to wrap the fish in foil or parchment paper, which essentially steams it. Another is to coat the fish lightly with flour, then bake it in a covered dish with a little fat-free stock or wine and your choice of herbs. These techniques are also suitable for shellfish.

Poultry preparation. Dredge skinless,

boneless pieces (breasts are leanest) in a little flour seasoned with ground black pepper. Then bake in a shallow dish with fat-free stock or wine, chopped fresh herbs (or crumbled dried ones) and chopped garlic.

Vegetables and fruit. Whole baked potatoes are perennial favourites – and much lower in fat than their roast and fried cousins. Instead of smothering them with butter, use low-fat sour cream or yogurt and chopped chives. For low-fat fries, cut potatoes into wedges, mist with non-stick spray and bake in a single layer until tender and browned.

Onions, carrots, peppers, courgettes, squash and aubergines also do well when baked, whether whole or in pieces. Baked peppers are excellent in salads and as side dishes. In sandwiches, they make mayonnaise unnecessary. Roast them whole at about 230°C/450°F/gas 8 until the skin blackens. It takes about 10 minutes on each side, but you need to check them every few minutes. (Alternatively, you can grill them, turning the peppers every 5 minutes.) Let them cool. Then halve, peel, remove the seeds and slice, or puree for spreading.

Baked garlic is a creamy substitute for butter on bread and baked potatoes and goes well with roast meat. Trim the tip of a garlic bulb to expose the cloves and wrap in foil. Roast at 150°C/375°F/gas 5 for about 30 minutes until the bulb softens. Cool slightly, then squeeze out the garlic.

Baked summer fruit (plums, apricots and peaches) make a great dessert with low-fat yogurt, Baked raisin-stuffed apples and pears can double as healthy side dishes for pork and poultry as well as for puddings.

Sweet stuff. Trim down your favourite cake and bread recipes by eliminating some of the fat and sugar. Start with one of the following suggestions. If that works to your satisfaction, incorporate another.

- Replace half the fat in a recipe with puréed fruit. Apple butter (which contains no butter) and puréed prunes both work well (see page 23 for recipe). For variety, try mashed cooked peaches or pears. Low-fat yogurt or buttermilk is also an option.

- Skimmed milk can take the place of full-fat.

- Nuts contain an amazing amount of calories and fat (although it's basically good, unsaturated fat). Cutting 6oz (175g) walnuts from a tea bread recipe saves you 385 calories and 37g of fat. When you do use nuts, give them a flavour boost by first toasting them (at 180°C/350°F/gas 4 for 5 minutes); then chop them finely for better dispersal.

- Use more raisins or other dried fruit to stand in for all or some of the nuts in tea breads and fruitcakes.

- Cut back on the amount of sugar in recipes. For every 7 oz (200g) you eliminate, you save 387 calories. A little ground cinnamon or nutmeg or a teaspoon of vanilla extract helps to compensate.

- Leave the bottom crust off fruit pies.

- Use two egg whites in place of a whole egg to save about 40 calories.

- Reduced-fat sour cream and cream cheese can easily replace their full-fat counterparts in cheesecakes.

- Grease baking tins with non-stick spray instead of butter, margarine or oil.

Roasting

Roasting is typically reserved for large pieces of meat. The beauty of roasting is its simplicity. You place food, such as a whole chicken or turkey, in the oven and don't fuss with it much until it's nearly done.

Simply succulent. For extra flavour, marinate meat, especially lower-fat cuts, before cooking and baste it as it roasts. Stock, wine, juice and low-fat vinegar-based salad dressings work well for both tasks. Slice off visible fat before cooking. Roast meat and poultry on a rack in a roasting pan to allow fat to drip off. Always roast poultry with the skin on to preserve moisture, but remove it before eating.

Vegetable magic. Roasting vegetables (effectively the same as baking – see page 92 – but with just a little fat) brings out their sweet, mellow flavours. Nearly any vegetable tastes great when roasted, even Jerusalem artichokes, asparagus, green beans, aubergines, cauliflower, broccoli and squash.

Lay out large chunks of vegetables in a single layer on a baking tray. Mist the vegetables with non-stick spray. Bake at 190°–220°C/375°–425°F/gas 5–7 until nicely browned, stirring the vegetables occasionally as they cook.

Braising

This slow, moist cooking method is perfect for the leanest cuts of meat and for hard vegetables like carrots and swede. Long, gentle cooking in a small amount of liquid turns sinewy meats into succulent treats and gives vegetables an extra measure of flavour.

The secret to successful braising is to simmer – not boil – the food. An oven set at 160°–180°C/325°–350°F/gas 2–4 is ideal, but you can also braise on the cooker top. Either way, a pot with a tight-fitting lid, such as a casserole dish, is essential.

Maximum flavour. The choice of liquid is key here. Water will suffice, but the dish will taste better with some or all fat-free stock, wine, fruit juice, or beer. You need enough liquid to cover about a third of the food. Enhance flavour with herbs and spices, fresh or dried.

Sear heaven. Braised meats are at their best when first seared in a hot frying pan. Searing browns the meat's surface, sealing in moisture. Searing also cooks off surface fat, which you should discard before continuing with the recipe.

A cooling break. After braising meat, allow it to cool in its liquid in the refrigerator for a few hours. The flavours blend and intensify, and the fat in the liquid rises to the top and hardens. Skim off that fat and say goodbye to 100 calories for every tablespoon you throw away. Reheat thoroughly in the oven or on the cooker

top, then serve.

Vegging out. Whole potatoes, carrots, onions, leeks and more can be braised, alone or along with meat. One pitfall to braising vegetables is that vitamins can escape into the cooking liquid. So use that liquid either as a sauce thickened with cornflour or as the basis for soup.

Grilling

Here, high heat sears the surface of food from the top.

Melting calories away. As food such as meat cooks, fat within it liquefies and drips through the rack into the grill pan. That's fat you won't be eating!

To increase flavour and tenderness, marinate meat and poultry before cooking. Acidic liquids like vinegar, fruit juice and wine do a great job.

Fish tales. The firmer the fish, the better it stands up to grilling. Tuna and swordfish steaks are very suitable. To prevent sticking, brush the grill with some olive oil or spritz it with non-stick spray before adding the fish.

Perfect produce. Most vegetables do best when grilled on foil, which stops them falling through the rack. Denser vegetables take longer to cook, so either cut them small or put them on the grill first.

Ears of sweetcorn, for instance, can be grilled in their husks. They'll be so sweet you won't even need butter. Kebabs are also perfect: skewer cherry tomatoes, chunks of pepper and whole mushrooms for colourful vegetable versions. Add small pieces of meat, chicken or whole prawns for a meal on a stick. For meatless burgers, grill mushroom caps and stack them on buns with reduced-fat cheese and tomato slices.

Fruit, including pineapple chunks and sliced peaches, pears and plums, may also be skewered and grilled. Or wrap larger pieces in foil and grill until soft. Either way, you have the makings of a sweet and refreshing starter, side dish or dessert.

Smart Seasonings

When food tastes great, there's no need to smother it with high-fat sauces. That's where herbs and spices come in. To get the most from them, keep these tips in mind.

Spice rack savvy. Dried herbs and spices, especially ground ones, have a limited shelf life. Keep an eye on best-before dates and throw out any that have gone musty or lost their smell.

A good basic set of herbs includes dried bay leaves, chilli powder, dill, oregano, paprika, sage, rosemary and thyme. Dried basil, chives and parsley are not very effective. Use fresh if you can. Useful spices include ground cinnamon, cloves, ginger and nutmeg. When you're feeling more adventurous, experiment with less familiar ones like cumin, coriander and Chinese five-spice powder.

The perfect pepper-upper. Purchase peppercorns whole and grind as needed to preserve their punch. Black peppercorns are all you really need, but a mixture of red, green, white and black will provide incomparable seasoning.

Fresh as a daisy. Dried herbs keep longer, but you can't beat the taste of fresh. Store in the refrigerator and wash just before use. To use, chop with a sharp knife or snip with kitchen shears. Keep fresh garlic on hand as well as fresh ginger (store the garlic in a cool, dry place and the ginger in the refrigerator).

While you're at it. Keep a range of vinegars including balsamic, raspberry, red wine, rice and malt. Vinegar's acidity tenderises meat while adding flavour. Vinegars with a distinctive flavour can actually let you cut calories in traditional vinaigrette dressings. Use up to half the usual oil quantity and make up the difference with vinegar. Pour the dressing into a water bottle with a spray attachment and mist salads lightly. (Herbs will clog the sprayer, so add them to the food separately.)

Extra-virgin olive oil is worth the expense. It's generally used for drizzling over fish, pasta, salads or fresh vegetables. Because of the cost you may not want to use it as a cooking oil. Yes, it's 100 per cent fat. But its flavour is so intense that you don't need to use much. Ditto for walnut oil and dark sesame oil.

Don't forget dehydrated sun-dried tomatoes to perk up pizzas and pasta dishes. Tomatoes packed in oil tend to taste better but contain extra calories.

Lemon and lime juice replace butter and margarine on steamed vegetables and add zip to fish and baked chicken. Fresh-squeezed is best.

Finally, don't banish salt from your table. Sometimes a light shake is all it takes to make low-fat food more palatable. Flavoured salts such as garlic and celery are useful, too.

Microwaving

The beauty of microwaving is that you don't need a trace of added fat to seal in flavours and nutrients.

The basics. Cooking time varies depending on a food's moisture content, how much you are cooking, the size of your dish and the power of your microwave, so keep checking on foods. You may remove foods when they are not quite done, since they continue to cook for a few minutes after they come out. If your oven doesn't have a turntable, rotate food so that it heats evenly.

Microwave mania. Vegetables and fruit are well-suited to low-fat microwave cookery. Whole potatoes, which normally take an hour or more to bake, can be microwaved in minutes. Pierce them with a fork first to allow steam to escape.

Chop other vegetables, such as broccoli, cauliflower, carrots and green beans, into uniform pieces. Place in a microwave-safe dish with about 1cm/½in of water, fat-free stock or wine. Cover with a piece of pierced plastic wrap. Cook on high power until just al dente.

Cored whole, halved or sliced fruits (especially apples and pears) can be microwaved successfully. Pop in some fruit while you're eating dinner, and your fat-free dessert will be ready when you are.

Fuss-free fare. Fish and chicken retain their tenderness when prepared in a microwave. Uniformity counts, however. Tuck the thin ends of a fish or chicken fillet underneath to ensure even cooking and moistness. Place in a dish with 1cm/½in of fat-free stock or wine and fresh chopped or dried herbs. Cover and microwave until just cooked through. Let stand a few minutes to finish cooking.

Microwaves don't brown meat, but you can cook minced beef, chicken breast or turkey breast to use in lasagne, chilli casseroles and spaghetti sauce. Crumble the meat into a glass bowl and microwave until no longer pink (stop and stir every two minutes). Drain the meat before using.

Steaming

This is a straightforward cooking method that, like microwaving, preserves taste and nutrients without added fat. It's an inexpensive technique, too, requiring only a collapsible steamer insert or a rack. (If you get into steaming big time, you can invest in an electric steamer or cooker top steamer pot.)

Gathering steam. Most vegetables are suitable for steaming. Cook only until crisp-tender to retain most flavour. Poultry, fish and shellfish work well, too. Pass up the traditional water in favour of fat-free stock, wine, beer or fruit juice. Add seasonings like herbs, spices and garlic. Use a pan that's big enough for the steam to circulate, and cover it with a tight lid. To steam fish, poultry, or vegetables in the oven, wrap them tightly in foil or parchment and bake at a high temperature (about 230°C/450°F/gas 8) for about 20 minutes, or until the food is tender.

Stir-Frying and Stir-Steaming

The two techniques of stir-frying and stir-steaming are identical, using a small amount of either oil or liquid to cook foods quickly. By combining bite-size pieces of meat, poultry or seafood with lots of low-calorie vegetables, you can make a little protein go a long way. And because foods cook so fast, they retain both flavour and nutrients.

Great beginnings. Prepare all your ingredients for stir-frying, including seasonings such as garlic, spring onions, fresh ginger and fresh chillis before starting to cook. Make sure your meat and vegetables are cut small so they cook fast. If desired, marinate the meat in a little low-salt soya sauce.

Next, get out a large non-stick frying pan or wok. A wok is helpful because it radiates heat quickly and evenly. Its rounded bottom and tall sides allow you to move food around fast without tossing it out of the pan. Coat the pan lightly with non-stick spray or a few pumps from a plastic bottle filled with corn or peanut oil (these oils won't burn over high heat). Heat the pan well. Leaving out the two tablespoons of oil typically used in stir-frying saves 240 calories right away.

Stir-steaming is simply stir-frying without the fat. Add a few tablespoons of water, fat-free stock, juice, wine or beer to the hot pan or wok before starting to cook your meat and vegetables in the same way.

A quick job. Once the pan is hot add the meat, poultry or seafood, limiting the amount to 90g (3oz) per serving. When it's almost cooked, add chopped garlic or pungent fresh chopped ginger and toss. Add chopped vegetables near the end to preserve their crispness. Try combinations of peppers, mangetout, broccoli, carrots, onions, mushrooms, cauliflower and asparagus. Cook until just crisp-tender. (It pays to steam denser veggies such as broccoli and carrots ahead of time so they're done at the same time as the tender ones.)

PART THREE

Body-Shaping Workouts

Chapter 8

Slim Your Waist and Flatten Your Tummy

Dawn MacInnes's waistline was absent without leave. As a teenager and in her twenties, Dawn was extremely active and had a tiny waist of 19–21in (47–52cm). But as she got older, her life changed – and so did her waistline, expanding to 28in (70cm). Now in her early forties, she has two children, aged five and nine.

'I had my first child at 31, and the second in my mid-thirties,' says Dawn, a trained nurse and sales representative for a medical technology company. 'I was also working full-time, sitting in an office. Then we moved house. Until we settled, we ate all our meals at hotels and in restaurants. On the job, I was in my car a lot and ate on the road. Between moving house, travelling and commuting, my diet went to pot.

'The weight I gained settled in areas where it had never settled before – my upper thighs and middle,' Dawn says. 'My skirts and jeans were tight. At first, I blamed it on the tumble drier. But then I got out of denial and realised that I had to do something or I'd have to buy all new clothes. And I'd be as big as a house by the time I reached 50.'

Previously, Dawn had tried walking to lose weight, but it didn't trim her waist the way she wanted. So she consulted Marjorie Albohm, an exercise physiologist, certified athletic trainer and director of sports medicine at a local city hospital. 'Marjorie gave me an extensive set of abdominal exercises targeted towards the middle, including curl-ups, crunches, side bends, hip raises and pelvic tilts. I do my ab exercises faithfully – as many as I can do in 30 minutes three or four days a week, either in the morning or evening. Plus, I walk for half-an-hour most afternoons, either outside or on a treadmill.'

Within three months, Dawn had regained her trim waistline of 22in (55cm).

'The results are incredible,' she says. 'I started to notice improvement in just a month. My waistbands started to feel comfortable. I tried on my jeans, and they fit again. My skirts weren't tight. In fact, they're a little loose now.'

Belly Be Gone

When it comes to bemoaning an expanding waistline, Dawn has lots of company. In a survey of more than 500 women conducted for this book, 67 per cent cited their bellies as trouble zones. Among the same women, 40 per cent named their waists as problem areas.

Your abdominal muscles confine your internal organs like a snug girdle. But pregnancy can present a challenge to these muscles. As a baby grows within the womb, the surrounding abdominal muscles – especially the lower abs – stretch . . . and stretch . . . and stretch. With each passing month, the muscle fibres lose strength and elasticity. If you have a second or third baby, the process repeats itself. If you have a caesarean delivery, in which the muscles are surgically separated, they become weaker still, losing their ability to expand and contract. When you add them up, these changes mean that your muscles lose their tone. The result is a post-pregnancy belly bulge.

Even if you've never been pregnant your tummy can protrude, especially when you approach menopause. Researchers aren't sure why, but the drop in female sex hormones that heralds menopause prompts fat to accumulate over your abs. If you're overweight all over, your abs may be temporarily obscured by an extra layer of fat.

Four Weeks to Tighter Abs

Anything that you can do to tighten your abdominal muscles will help hold in your stomach and other organs. Your abs consist of four muscles, all of which shape your torso.

- The rectus abdominis (upper and lower), a vertical muscle that runs from your ribcage to your pubic bone
- The transverse abdominis, the deepest ab, which runs horizontally across your torso
- The external oblique, a broad, thin muscle that runs diagonally from your ribs to your hip
- The internal oblique muscle, which runs along the front and sides of your torso

The upper and lower abs and the obliques are 'helper' muscles: you can press them into service as needed. If you're lying on your back on the beach and you reach forward to apply sunscreen to your knees, you're working your upper abs. If you're lying on the floor watching TV and you raise your legs, you're working your lower abs. If you're standing at the office photocopier and you bend to the right or left, you're working your obliques.

The trouble is, we don't routinely tax our abs very much during the course of a day. If we worked them harder, or more often, or both, they would tighten up and get stronger, and our tummies wouldn't protrude.

To slim your waist and a tummy distended by pregnancy, surplus weight or hormonal changes, you need a programme of exercises that deliberately works the abs – especially the

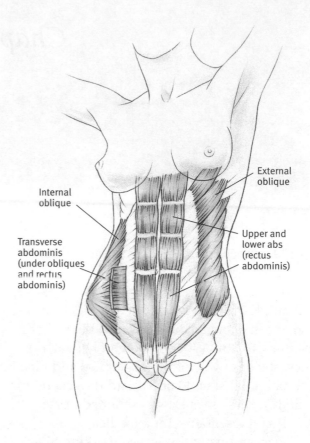

Internal oblique

External oblique

Transverse abdominis (under obliques and rectus abdominis)

Upper and lower abs (rectus abdominis)

To slim your waist and flatten your stomach, you need to work the upper and lower abs and the oblique muscles in the abdominal area.

upper and lower abs and the obliques – as well as a weight-loss regime to lose excess fat. Working the abs as you go about your daily duties helps, too. The torso-shaping workouts that follow show you how.

'Like Dawn, you may see results in as little as four weeks,' says Marjorie Albohm, who works with women ranging from beginners who've never broken a sweat to highly trained fitness enthusiasts.

'The abdominal muscles are wonderful to work on because they respond very quickly to exercise,' says Albohm. 'Compared to your buttocks, thighs or other muscle groups, the abs get stronger pretty quickly.'

The workouts that follow produce results because they use the principle of overload: they boost muscular effort by increasing either duration (by doing more repetitions) or intensity (by doing the same number of reps but adding weights to make the exercise harder). If you're new to exercise, start at the beginner level. Once you can complete the programme with relative ease for three consecutive workout sessions, it's time to progress to the next level.

'You'll feel results in about two weeks,' says Albohm. 'By four weeks, you should see some tightening or slight changes in contour. And by six weeks, you'll look and feel toned. If you don't, you're not doing the exercises correctly.'

Maximum Results with Minimum Effort

To make sure you get results, Albohm suggests doing these torso-shaping workouts in front of a mirror so you can check your position. 'If you've never exercised before, you may have no idea what position your head, neck, shoulders and back are in, or how far off the floor you are.'

Here are some other tips from Albohm for getting the fastest results with the least effort.

Work all the abs. If you're trying to regain muscle tone after pregnancy, you will probably want to focus more on the lower abs. But don't neglect the others. As a rule, you should work the upper and lower abs and the obliques equally.

Flex those knees. If you don't, you're likely to use your hip muscles, not your abs, which will defeat the purpose of the exercise. As you advance, you may be doing straight-leg raises.

Flatten your back. You should flatten your back against the floor to protect your lower back muscles against strain. Use an exercise mat, carpeted floor or large, folded towel.

Start easy. Three to 10 repetitions is the maximum for beginners.

Use slow, controlled movements. Do this, and hold each position for a count of two, suggests Albohm. If you experience pain or discomfort when performing an exercise, stop and substitute another version, she advises. If pain persists, see your doctor.

Be consistent. 'Next to performing the exercises correctly, exercising regularly is key,' says Albohm. The beginner, intermediate and experienced workouts outlined on the following pages should be done three or four times a week. Use the everyday version that's shown with some of the exercises to work the same muscles in your daily life.

Combine ab work with diet and aerobics. 'You can't say, "I want to take 3in (75cm) off my waist", do 500 ab exercises and nothing else, and expect it to work – it won't,' says Albohm. If you ignore aerobic exercise – and a sensible diet – your belly will show it.

Combining aerobics with ab workouts helps in two ways: the combination burns calories, which helps get rid of excess weight all over, including the abdomen, and it gives your abs a little boost.

'The fact that you're supporting your body as you move forces the muscles to contract,' explains Albohm. 'If you deliberately contract your abs during aerobic exercise, you'll benefit even more.'

Be patient. 'Don't expect results overnight,' says Albohm.

CURL-UPS 1

Muscles worked
Upper abs

Performance hints

- Use your abs to do the work. Don't pull yourself up with your arms.
- Keep your back flat on the floor.

Intensity

Beginner: 1 set of 3–10 reps, 3 days per week

Intermediate: 2 sets of 10 reps, 3 days per week

Experienced: 3 or 4 sets of 10 reps, 3 or 4 days per week

Everyday version for upper abs

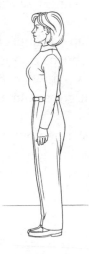

While standing, contract your upper abdominals by inhaling sharply and holding in your abdominal muscles. Breathing normally, hold for 6–8 seconds, then release.

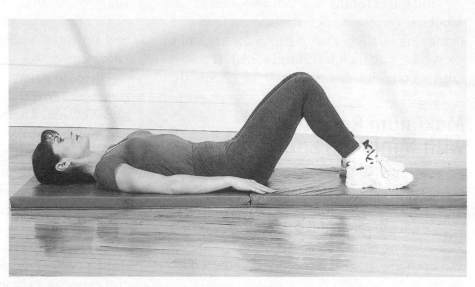

LIE ON YOUR BACK with your pelvis tilted to flatten your back against the floor, arms at your sides, knees bent at approximately a 90-degree angle, and your feet flat on the floor.

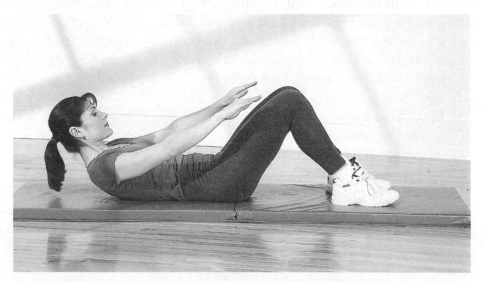

USING YOUR UPPER abdominal muscles, raise your head and shoulders from the floor. Your arms should be extended in front. Hold for 2 seconds. Then lower your shoulders to the floor in a slow, controlled motion, touching your shoulders lightly on the floor. Repeat.

CURL-UPS 2

Muscles worked
Upper abs

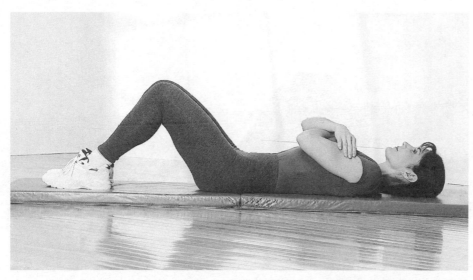

LIE ON YOUR BACK with your pelvis tilted to flatten your back, arms folded across your chest, knees bent approximately 90 degrees, and your feet flat on the floor.

Performance hints

- Keep your feet and lower back flat on the floor.
- Don't rock, using the momentum to pull yourself up.
- Don't strain your head or neck when rising.

Intensity

Beginner: 1 set of 3–10 reps, 3 days per week

Intermediate: 2 sets of 10 reps, 3 days per week

Experienced: 3 or 4 sets of 10 reps, 3 or 4 days per week

Variation

To increase intensity further, you can hold a 1-lb (0.5-kg) dumbbell on your chest while performing this curl-up. For still more intensity, add up to 3lb (1.5kg).

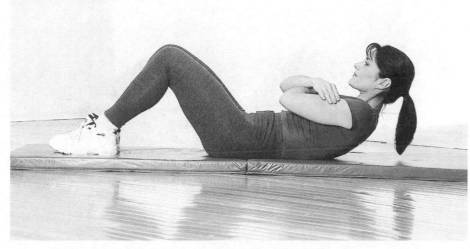

USING YOUR UPPER abdominal muscles, raise your head and shoulders from the floor towards your knees. Hold for 2 seconds. Then lower your upper body in a slow, controlled motion, touching your shoulders lightly on the floor. Repeat.

CURL-UPS 3

Muscles worked

Upper abs

Performance hints

■ Don't pull your head and neck upwards when lifting your shoulders.

■ To prevent neck strain, keep your chin forwards and your eyes focused towards the ceiling.

■ Keep your elbows out to your sides so you can barely see them.

Intensity

Beginner: 1 set of 3–10 reps, 3 days per week

Intermediate: 2 sets of 10 reps, 3 days per week

Experienced: 3 or 4 sets of 10 reps, 3 or 4 days per week

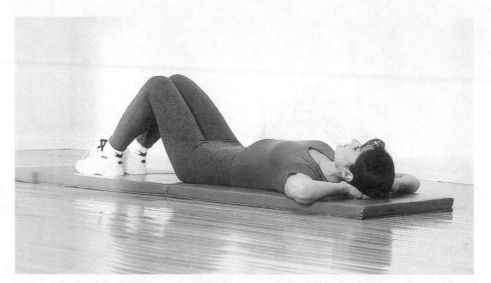

LIE ON YOUR BACK with your pelvis tilted to flatten your back, your knees bent at approximately 90 degrees, and your hands clasped behind your head. Your elbows should be out to your sides, and your feet flat on the floor.

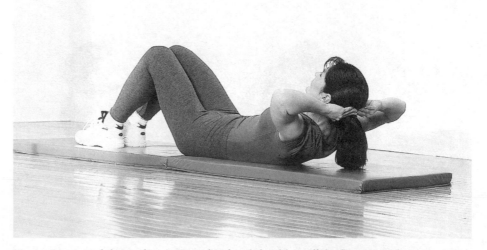

USING YOUR UPPER abdominals, raise your head and shoulders off the floor. Hold for 2 seconds. Then lower your upper body to the floor in a slow, controlled motion, touching your shoulders lightly on the floor. Repeat.

KNEE-UP CRUNCHES

Muscles worked
Upper abs

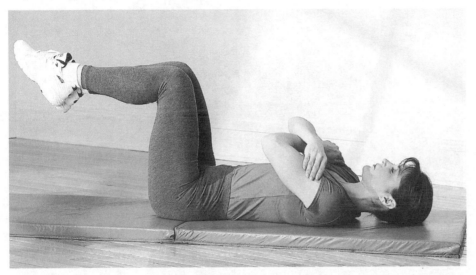

LIE ON YOUR BACK with your legs raised so that your thighs are perpendicular to your body and your calves and feet are parallel to the floor. Fold your arms across your chest.

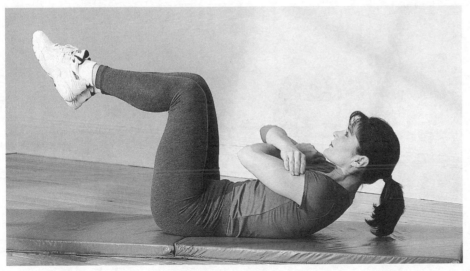

USING THE MUSCLES of your upper abs, raise your shoulders and upper back off the floor in a forward curling motion. Hold for 2 seconds. Then slowly lower your shoulders to the starting position, lightly touching them to the floor. Repeat.

Performance hints

- Make sure that your shoulders lift off the floor.
- Don't use momentum to perform the move.
- Keep the small of your back pressed against the floor.

Intensity

Beginner: 1 set of 3–10 reps, 3 days per week

Intermediate: 2 sets of 10 reps, 3 days per week

Experienced: 3 or 4 sets of 10 reps, 3 or 4 days per week

Variation

To increase intensity further, you can hold a 1-lb (0.5-kg) dumbbell on your chest while performing this crunch. For still more intensity, use 2lb (1kg).

Everyday version for upper abs

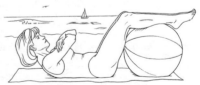

You can simulate this exercise while lying on the beach or your living room floor with your legs propped up by a beach ball.

CRUNCHES WITH KNEES UP, SPREAD

Muscles worked
Upper abs

Performance hints

- Keep the movement slow and controlled.

- Don't pull your head or neck with your hands as you go up.

- Don't rest your shoulders on the floor at the bottom of the movement.

Intensity

Beginner: 1 set of 3–10 reps, 3 days per week

Intermediate: 2 sets of 10 reps, 3 days per week

Experienced: 3 or 4 sets of 10 reps, 3 or 4 days per week

Everyday version for upper abs

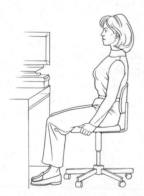

While sitting at your desk, contract your upper abdominals by inhaling sharply and pulling in your abdominal area. Breathing normally, hold for 6–8 seconds, then relax. Repeat.

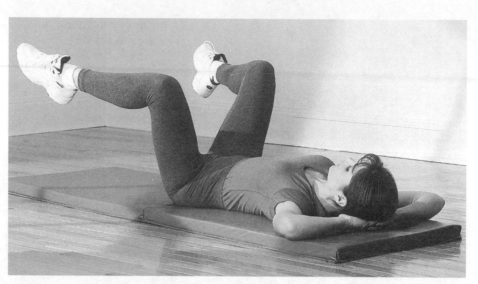

LYING ON YOUR BACK, raise your legs so your thighs are perpendicular to your body, with your calves and feet raised and parallel to the floor, and your hands behind your head with your elbows extended. Spread your legs.

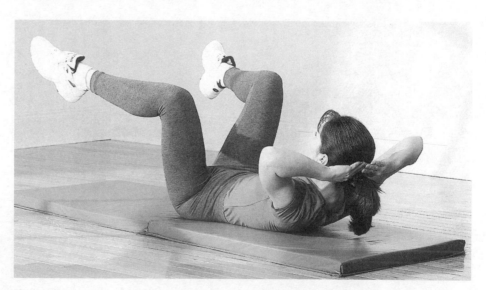

USING YOUR UPPER ABS, raise your shoulders and upper back off the floor in a slow, controlled forward curling motion. Hold for 2 seconds. Then lower your shoulders to the starting position, lightly touching them to the floor. Repeat.

INCLINED BOARD CRUNCHES

Muscles worked
Upper abs

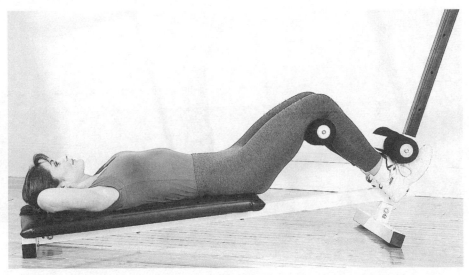

LIE FLAT ON YOUR BACK on an inclined board with your feet hooked under the footrest and your hands behind your head, with your elbows extended.

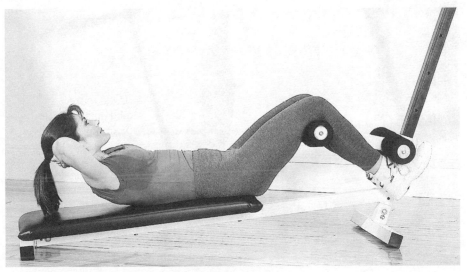

USING YOUR UPPER ABS, raise your head and shoulders off the bench in a forward curling motion. Hold for 2 seconds. Then lower your shoulders in a slow, controlled motion to the starting position, lightly touching them to the bench. Repeat.

Performance hints

- Don't use your hands to pull up on your head and neck.
- Don't relax at the bottom of the movement.

Intensity

Beginner: 1 set of 3–10 reps, 3 days per week

Intermediate: 2 sets of 10 reps, 3 days per week

Experienced: 3 or 4 sets of 10 reps, 3 or 4 days per week

Variation

You can increase the intensity by increasing the angle of the bench.

Everyday version for upper abs

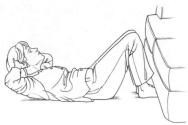

You can simulate this exercise by performing it with your feet hooked underneath a very heavy, secure piece of furniture.

HIP RAISES

Muscles worked
Lower abs

Performance hints

- Don't use your arms or shoulders to assist in the lift.
- Don't rock your hips backwards.
- Don't let your legs fall backwards towards your head.

Intensity

Beginner: 1 set of 3–10 reps, 3 days per week

Intermediate: 2 sets of 10 reps, 3 days per week

Experienced: 3 or 4 sets of 10 reps, 3 or 4 days per week

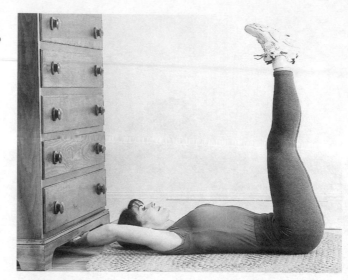

LIE ON YOUR BACK with your legs extended upwards, toes pointed, and your arms extended overhead. Hold on to a heavy, secure piece of furniture such as the bottom of a chest or sofa.

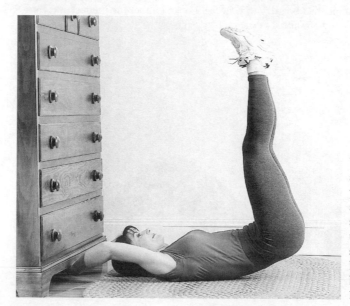

USING YOUR LOWER abdominal muscles, raise your hips off the floor and lift your legs, knees slightly flexed, straight in the air. Hold for 2 seconds. Then lower your legs, touching your hips lightly on the floor. Repeat.

MODIFIED KNEE RAISES

Muscles worked
Lower abs

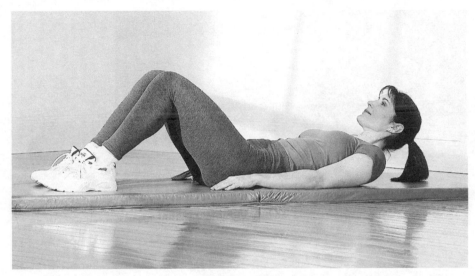

Performance hints

- Keep the opposite foot on the floor.
- Don't raise your head and neck too much; your shoulder blades should be only slightly off the floor.

Intensity

Beginner: 1 set of 3–10 reps, 3 days per week

Intermediate: 2 sets of 10 reps, 3 days per week

Experienced: 3 or 4 sets of 10 reps, 3 or 4 days per week

LIE ON YOUR BACK with your pelvis tilted to flatten your back and your knees bent. Your arms should be extended next to your body with your hands palms down, your head up, and your shoulder blades slightly off the floor.

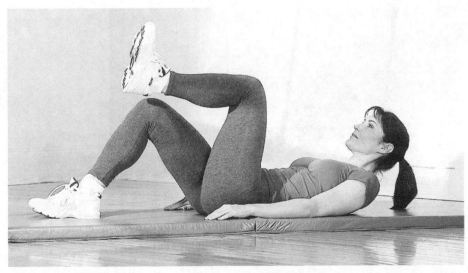

USING YOUR LOWER abdominals, raise one leg at a time towards your chest in a slow, controlled motions. Hold for 2 seconds. Then lower your leg slowly until your heel lightly touches the floor. Repeat with the opposite leg.

PELVIC TILTS

Muscles worked
Lower abs

Performance hint

■ Don't raise your head and neck off the floor.

Intensity

Beginner: 1 set of 3–10 reps, 3 days per week

Intermediate: 2 sets of 10 reps, 3 days per week

Experienced: 3 or 4 sets of 10 reps, 3 or 4 days per week

Everyday version for lower abs

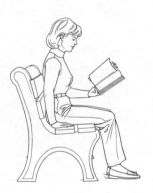

While sitting, perform the same exercise by slightly tilting your pelvis up, contracting your lower abdominals and slightly pushing your lower back flat. Hold for 8–10 seconds, then release.

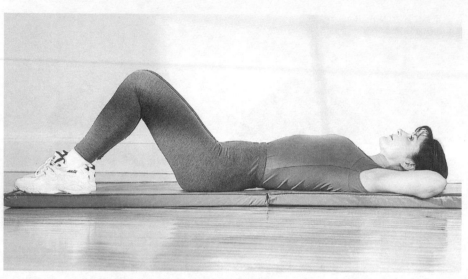

LIE FLAT ON YOUR BACK with your knees bent at approximately a 90-degree angle and your hands behind your head, elbows extended to your sides, and your head on the floor.

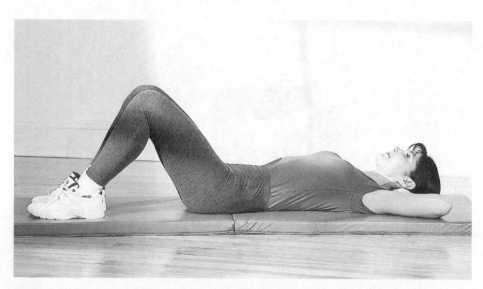

LIFT YOUR PELVIS UP and towards your ribcage, tightening your lower abdominal muscles and gently 'pushing' back into the floor. Hold for 2 seconds. Relax and let your pelvis rotate back to its normal position. Repeat the exercise in a slow, controlled manner.

REVERSE CURLS

Muscles worked
Lower abs

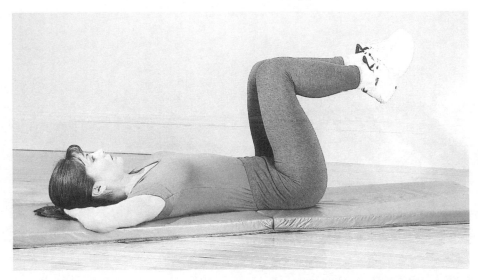

LIE FLAT ON YOUR BACK with your head flat on the floor, your hands behind your head supporting your neck, and your elbows out. Raise your legs so that your thighs are perpendicular to your body, and your calves and feet are parallel to the floor.

Performance hints

- Don't rock or use momentum to perform the curl.
- Don't rest your hips on the floor at the bottom of the curl.
- Keep constant tension on your abs during the exercise.

Intensity

Beginner: 1 set of 3–10 reps, 3 days per week

Intermediate: 2 sets of 10 reps, 3 days per week

Experienced: 3 or 4 sets of 10 reps, 3 or 4 days per week

Variation

To increase intensity, straighten your lower legs slightly as you perform the exercise.

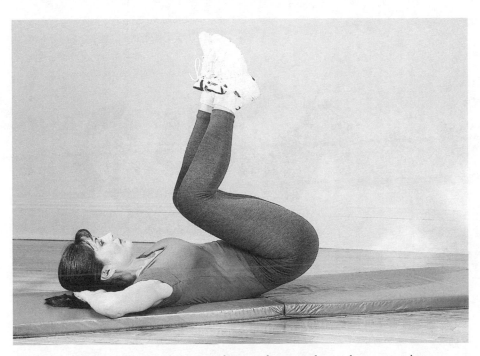

USING YOUR LOWER ABS, raise your hips towards your ribcage, with your knees towards your forehead. Hold for a count of 2. Then lower your hips in a slow, controlled motion, keeping your abs contracted until your hips contact the floor. Repeat.

SINGLE-KNEE LIFTS

Muscles worked
Upper and lower abs

Performance hints

- When rising, don't pull on your head and neck with your arms.
- Raise your torso and knees together in an equidistant curling motion.
- Don't use momentum to rock upwards.

Intensity

Beginner: 1 set of 3–10 reps on each side, 3 days per week

Intermediate: 2 sets of 10 reps on each side, 3 days per week

Experienced: 3 or 4 sets of 10 reps on each side, 3 or 4 days per week

Everyday version for upper and lower abs

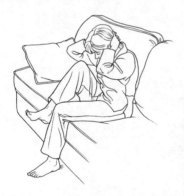

While sitting, place your hands behind your head. With one foot flat on the floor, bring the opposite knee up to meet your torso. Contract your upper abdominals as you crunch forward to meet your raised knee; hold for 8–10 seconds. Return your upper body and leg in a slow, controlled motion. Repeat with the opposite leg. Repeat the exercise using your lower abdominals.

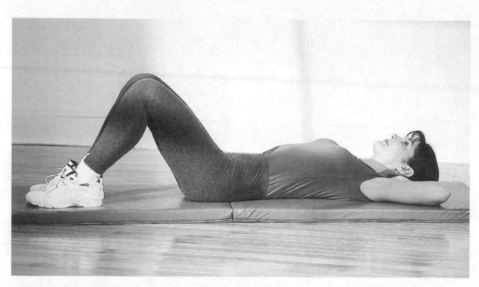

LIE ON YOUR BACK with your knees bent, your feet on the floor, and your pelvis tilted to flatten your back. Your hands should be behind your head and your elbows extended.

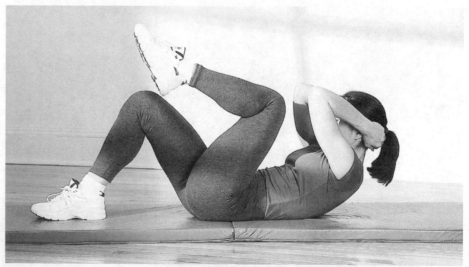

USING YOUR UPPER and lower abs, simultaneously raise one knee and your torso, bringing both elbows to the knee. Hold for 2 seconds. Then lower your upper body and leg in a slow, controlled motion. Repeat on the opposite side.

DIAGONAL CURL-UPS 1

Muscles worked
Obliques

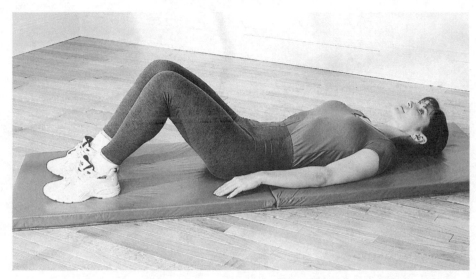

LIE ON YOUR BACK with your feet flat on the floor, your knees bent at approximately a 90-degree angle, your pelvis tilted to flatten your back, and your arms straight at your sides.

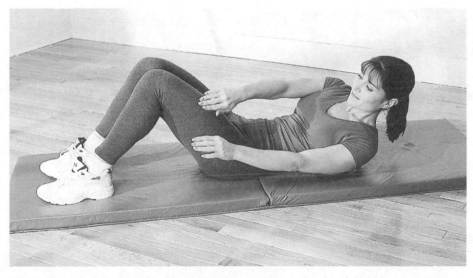

EXTEND YOUR ARMS and use your oblique muscles to raise your head and shoulders, rotating to one side as your shoulders lift off the floor. Hold for 2 seconds. Then lower your shoulders in a slow, controlled motion, touching them lightly to the floor. Repeat the exercise on the opposite side.

Performance hints

■ Don't use your arms to pull up your shoulders.

■ As you rotate your torso, use a slow, controlled motion and keep your oblique muscles contracted.

■ Don't use momentum to alternate from side to side.

Intensity

Beginner: 1 set of 3–10 reps on each side, 3 days per week

Intermediate: 2 sets of 10 reps on each side, 3 days per week

Experienced: 3 or 4 sets of 10 reps on each side, 3 or 4 days per week

Everyday version for obliques

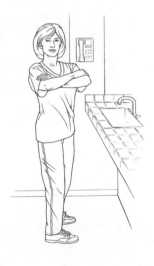

While standing at the kitchen sink or a photocopier, rotate your upper body one quarter turn in a slow, controlled motion. Fold your arms and contract your abdominal muscles while turning. Hold for 6–8 seconds, then repeat the exercise for the opposite side.

DIAGONAL CURL-UPS 2

Muscles worked
Obliques

Performance hints

- Keep your feet flat on the floor.
- Don't use momentum when rotating from side to side.
- Don't over-rotate.

Intensity

Beginner: 1 set of 3–10 reps on each side, 3 days per week

Intermediate: 2 sets of 10 reps on each side, 3 days per week

Experienced: 3 or 4 sets of 10 reps on each side, 3 or 4 days per week

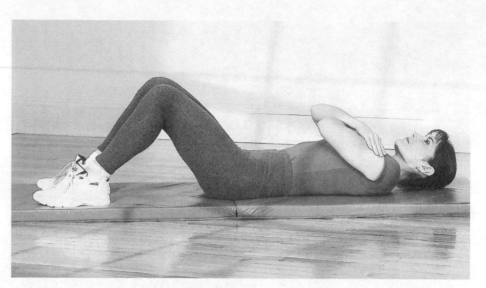

LIE ON YOUR BACK with your pelvis tilted to flatten your back against the floor, your knees bent at approximately a 90-degree angle, your feet flat on the floor, and your arms folded across your chest.

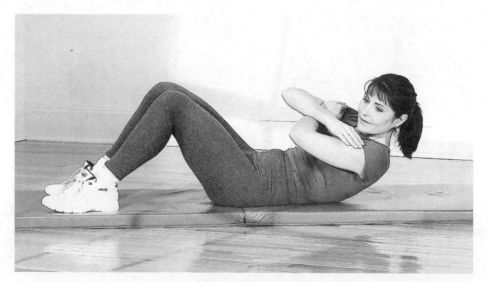

USE YOUR OBLIQUE MUSCLES to raise your head and shoulders from the floor, rotating to one side as your shoulders lift off the floor. Hold for 2 seconds. Lower your shoulders in a slow, controlled motion, touching them lightly to the floor. Repeat the exercise in the opposite direction.

DIAGONAL CURL-UPS 3

Muscles worked
Obliques

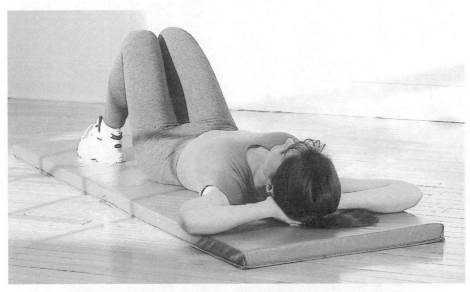

Performance hints
- Don't pull on your head and neck.
- Don't over-rotate.
- Don't use momentum when alternating sides.

Intensity

Beginner: 1 set of 3–10 reps on each side, 3 days per week

Intermediate: 2 sets of 10 reps on each side, 3 days per week

Experienced: 3 or 4 sets of 10 reps on each side, 3 or 4 days per week

LIE ON YOUR BACK with your feet flat on the floor and your knees bent at approximately 90 degrees, with your pelvis tilted to flatten your back. Your hands should be clasped behind your head with your elbows out to your sides.

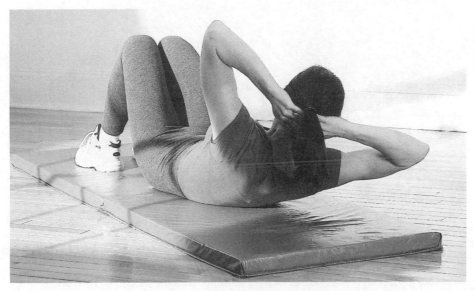

USE YOUR OBLIQUE MUSCLES to raise your head and shoulders, rotating to one side as your shoulders lift off the floor. Hold for 2 seconds. Then lower your shoulders in a slow, controlled motion, touching them lightly to the floor. Repeat the exercise in the opposite direction.

SIDE CRUNCHES

Muscles worked
Obliques

Performance hints

- Make sure your upper body is lifted off the floor, not just your head and neck.
- Don't pull on your head and neck with your hand.
- Feel the muscle contraction in the oblique area.

Intensity

Beginner: 1 set of 3–10 reps on each side, 3 days per week

Intermediate: 2 sets of 10 reps on each side, 3 days per week

Experienced: 3 or 4 sets of 10 reps on each side, 3 or 4 days per week

Everyday version for obliques

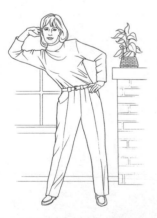

Stand with your feet comfortably apart. Place your right arm behind your head with your elbow extended, and the other arm on your hip. Using your oblique muscles, flex your trunk to the right side. Hold for 6–8 seconds, then relax. Repeat on the opposite side.

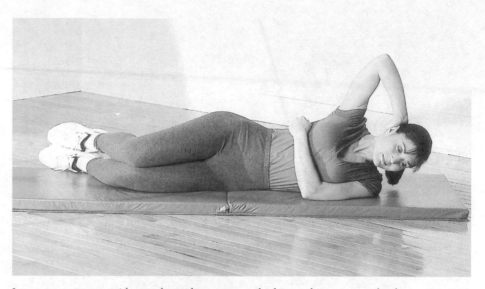

LIE ON YOUR LEFT HIP, with your knees bent so your thighs are almost perpendicular to your body. Place your right hand behind your head, elbow extended, and your left hand on top of your right side.

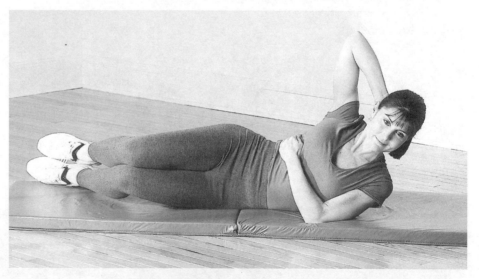

USING YOUR OBLIQUE MUSCLES in a crunchlike motion, lift your upper body off the floor and up over your hip, bringing your ribcage towards your hip. Hold for 2 seconds. Then lower your body in a slow, controlled motion, slightly touching the floor. Repeat the movement on the same side until you have completed your repetitions. Then perform the same exercise on the opposite side.

SIDE BENDS

Muscles worked
Obliques

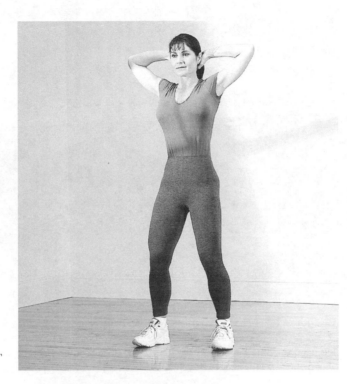

STAND WITH YOUR KNEES slightly bent, feet shoulder-width apart, hands behind your head, and elbows extended.

Performance hints

- Perform the movement in a slow and controlled manner throughout a full range of motion.
- Don't use momentum when performing repetitions.
- Don't lean forward as you bend.

Intensity

Beginner: 1 set of 3–10 reps on each side, 3 days per week

Intermediate: 2 sets of 10 reps on each side, 3 days per week

Experienced: 3 or 4 sets of 10 reps on each side, 3 or 4 days per week

Everyday version for obliques

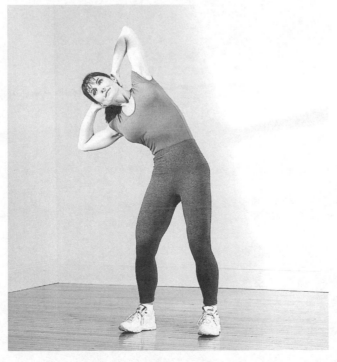

USING YOUR OBLIQUE muscles, bend to your right side in a slow, controlled movement, bringing your right elbow towards your right knee. Return to the starting position and repeat the movement on the same side until you have completed your repetitions. Perform the same exercise on the opposite side.

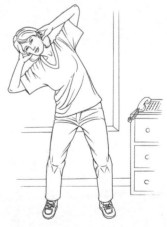

Stand with your feet comfortably apart in a quarter-squat position with your hands behind your head and your elbows extended. Using your oblique muscles, bend to one side approximately 25–30 degrees. Hold for 6–8 seconds, then relax. Repeat on the opposite side.

SIDE JACK-KNIVES

Muscles worked
Obliques

Performance hints

- Lift both your upper and lower body an equal distance.
- Perform the exercise in a slow, controlled motion; don't use momentum.
- Make sure you lift your upper body off the floor, not just your head.

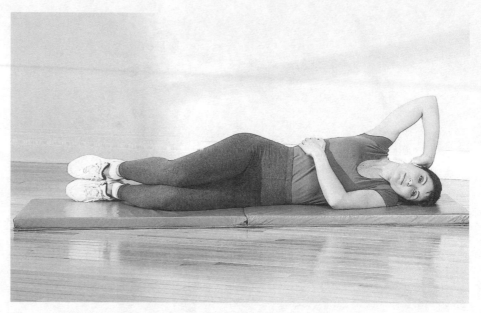

LIE ON YOUR LEFT SIDE with your legs together, your knees bent, and your thighs almost perpendicular to your body. Your left arm should be close to your body for support, with your left hand on your waist. Your right hand should be on the side of your head, with elbow bent.

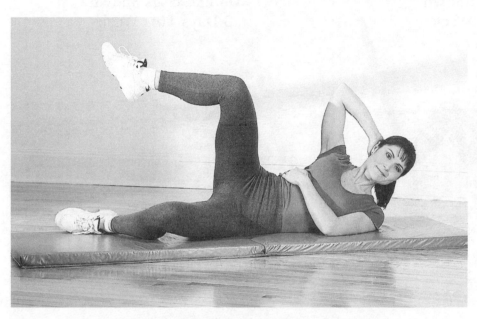

Intensity

Beginner: 1 set of 3–10 reps on each side, 3 days per week

Intermediate: 2 sets of 10 reps on each side, 3 days per week

Experienced: 3 or 4 sets of 10 reps on each side, 3 or 4 days per week

USING YOUR OBLIQUE MUSCLES, raise your top leg while simultaneously raising your head, shoulders and torso. Hold for 2 seconds. Then lower in a controlled motion. After completing your repetitions, repeat on the opposite side.

30-DAY BEGINNER PROGRAMME

Week 1

**Do Exercises Shown
3 Days This Week**

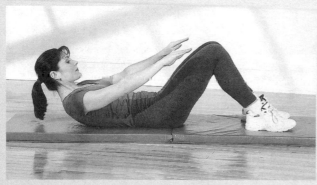

Curl-Ups 1 (page 102)

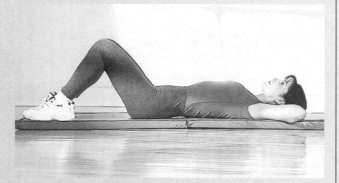

Pelvic Tilts (page 110)

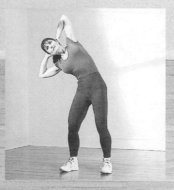

Side Bends (page 117)

Week 2

**Do Exercises Shown
3 Days This Week**

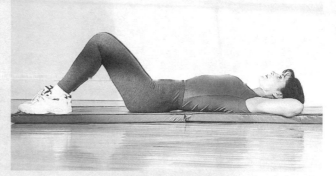

Pelvic Tilts (page 110)

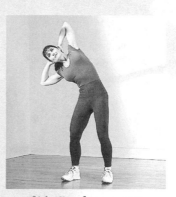

Side Bends (page 117)

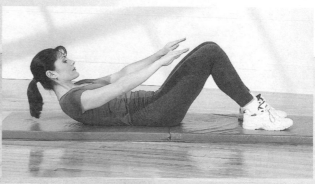

Curl-Ups 1 (page 102)

Week 3

Do Exercises Shown
3 Days This Week

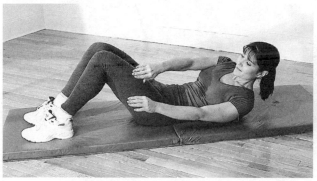

Diagonal Curl-Ups 1 (page 113)

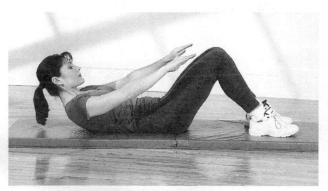

Curl-Ups 1 (page 102)

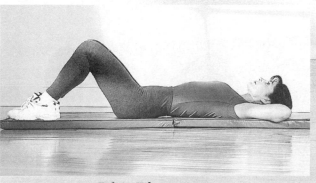

Pelvic Tilts (page 110)

Week 4

Do Exercises Shown
3 Days This Week

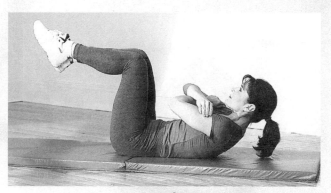

Knee-Up Crunches (page 105)

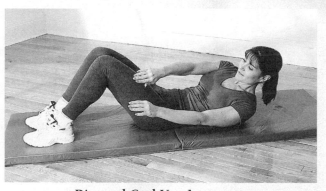

Diagonal Curl-Ups 1 (page 113)

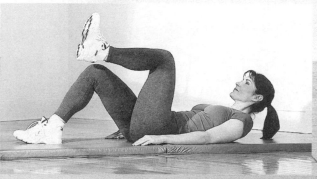

Modified Knee Raises (page 109)

30-Day Intermediate Programme

Week 1	**Week 2**
Do Exercises Shown 3 Days This Week	Do Exercises Shown 3 Days This Week

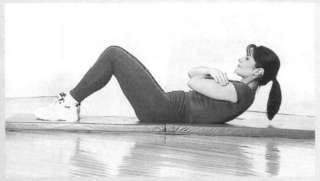

Curl-Ups 2 (page 103)

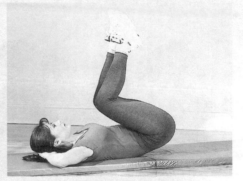

Reverse Curls (page 111)

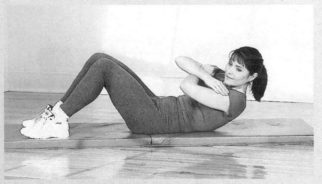

Diagonal Curl-Ups 2 (page 114)

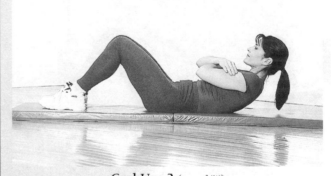

Curl-Ups 2 (page 103)

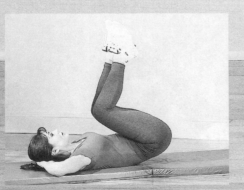

Reverse Curls (page 111)

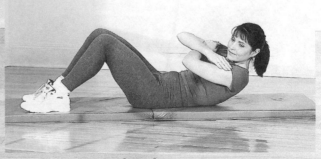

Diagonal Curl-Ups 2 (page 114)

Week 3

Do Exercises Shown
3 Days This Week

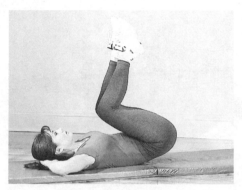

Reverse Curls (page 111)

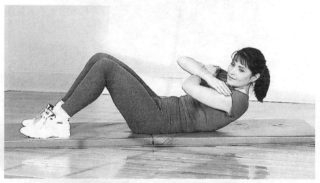

Diagonal Curl-Ups 2 (page 114)

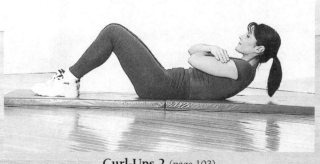

Curl-Ups 2 (page 103)

Week 4

Do Exercises Shown
3 Days This Week

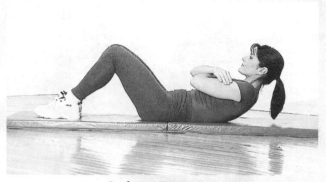

Curl-Ups 2 (page 103)

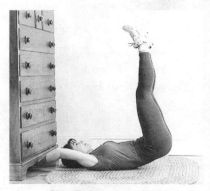

Hip Raises (page 108)

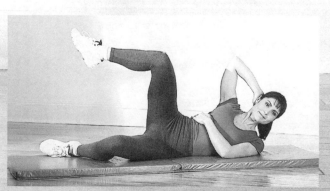

Side Jack-knives (page 118)

30-Day Experienced Programme

Week 1

**Do Exercises Shown
3 or 4 Days This Week**

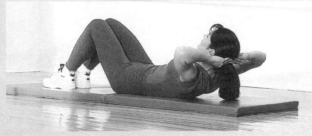

Curl-Ups 3 (page 104)

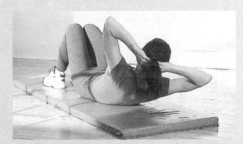

Diagonal Curl-Ups 3 (page 115)

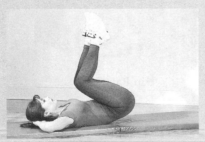

Reverse Curls (page 111)

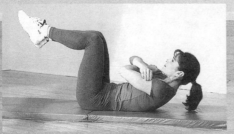

Knee-Up Crunches (page 105)

Week 2

**Do Exercises Shown
3 or 4 Days This Week**

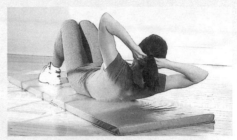

Diagonal Curl-Ups 3 (page 115)

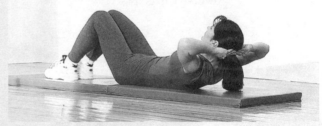

Curl-Ups 3 (page 104)

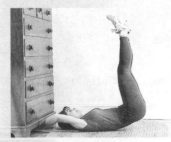

Hip Raises (page 108)

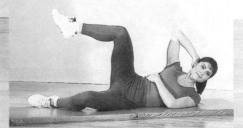

Side Jack-knives (page 118)

Week 3

Do Exercises Shown
3 or 4 Days This Week

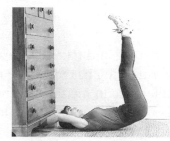

Hip Raises (page 108)

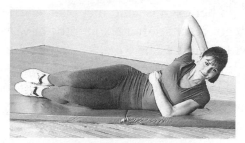

Side Crunches (page 116)

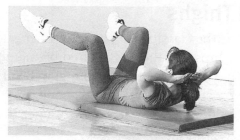

Crunches with Knees Up, Spread (page 106)

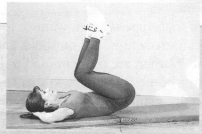

Reverse Curls (page 111)

Week 4

Do Exercises Shown
3 or 4 Days This Week

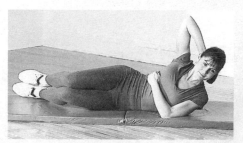

Side Crunches (page 116)

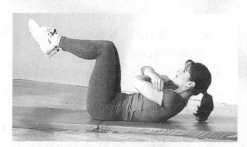

Knee-Up Crunches (page 105)

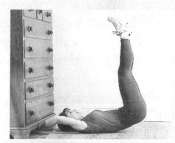

Hip Raises (page 108)

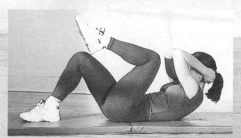

Single-Knee Lifts (page 112)

Chapter 9

Workouts for Your Hips, Thighs and Buttocks

By many women's standards, Carrie wasn't what you would call overweight. Before she had children, she weighed a mere 7 stone 2lb (45kg). Even at the age of 43, petite (5ft 1in/1.5m) Carrie weighed just 8 stone 5lb (53kg). Problem was, the extra weight seemed to have accumulated on her hips and thighs.

'I was definitely pear-shaped,' says Carrie, an art teacher with three teenage daughters. Like many pear-shaped women, Carrie couldn't find jeans and trousers to fit her proportions. 'I'd find a pair that fit in the hips, but the waist would be too big. If I found a pair that fit in the waist, I couldn't get them over my thighs. I'd try on 20 pairs, but I still couldn't find any that looked stylish and felt comfortable.'

Carrie blamed heredity, having children and her age. She tried to lose weight by cutting out certain foods entirely, not eating altogether and following 'diets' she improvised. She also tried running and swimming, but she wasn't very consistent. She just couldn't trim her hips and thighs – until she started to work out with weights.

'My sister runs a fitness centre, and she encouraged me to try weight training,' says Carrie. 'I started to work out, doing leg raises, curls, extensions and especially lunges three days a week. I lost inches on my hips and thighs, but especially my thighs.'

In addition Carrie spends time on a step machine, for 5–15 minutes a session, or she does a 40-minute aerobic class to warm up. And she's more consistent about aerobic exercise. 'I run, bike and take aerobics classes. But the weight training has made the most significant difference in my thighs,' she says.

Carrie also follows a more structured low-fat diet, which includes lots of fruit, vegetables, cereal and soya milk. For protein, she eats fish and tofu, and a little red meat.

With her exercise and diet plan, Carrie finally got results. After six months of working out with weights, she weighs 7 stone 12lb (50kg). But to Carrie, the important thing is that she lost fat and gained muscle (and more energy). And she finally found jeans to fit and look good.

Thinner, Shapelier Hips and Thighs

Carrie is the classic pear shape and her quest for thinner hips and thighs is shared by many women, young and not-so-young. In a survey of 500 women conducted for this book, nearly half said they wished they had slimmer thighs and over 40 per cent said they were dissatisfied with their hips. A fair number – 25 per cent – also said they regarded their backsides as a trouble zone.

It's not that these women want to look like men, with narrow hips, flat buttocks and wide shoulders. Women are programmed to have wider lower bodies than men so that they can cope with pregnancy and childbearing.

In some women, this pear shape is particularly exaggerated, even if they're only a little overweight. This makes it hard to find even 'easy-fit' jeans that are comfortable, and it makes women self-conscious about wearing swimsuits.

Heavier hips, thighs and buttocks are more a factor of gender than of age. 'Whether they're 20 or 40, women still have 10–15 per cent more body fat than men, even if they work out,' says Albohm. As for the myth that pregnancy 'stretches' your pelvis and widens your hips, that's just not so, says exercise physiologist, Marjorie Albohm. 'If women have bigger hips after pregnancy they've simply gained weight, full stop.'

Nor is sitting at a desk responsible for wider hips and a broader backside. 'Sitting itself doesn't necessarily determine where fat is deposited,' says Albohm. 'Our sedentary lifestyle in general does that. Your muscles would be far more toned if you were active – working on a farm, climbing up and down ladders and so forth. Those are the exercises that tone the muscles in your hips and thighs.'

Done correctly, cutting dietary fat and calories can help you lose weight overall, and that can certainly help 'shrink' your hips, thighs and buttocks to some degree. So can aerobic exercise that burns excess body fat and calories as you work your heart and lungs, like walking, jogging, cycling or taking aerobics classes. Purposeful exercise can make up for the kind of sedentary lifestyle that packs pounds on everywhere, including the hips and thighs. But to see a real difference in your lower body, says Albohm, you have to do what Carrie did – add resistance training to the mix.

Muscles Meant to Be Worked

The muscles of the hips, thighs and buttocks include:

- The gluteal muscles (small, medium and large muscles that form the buttocks)
- The quadriceps (the muscles on the front of the thighs)
- The hamstrings (the muscles on the back of the thighs)
- The abductors (the outer thighs)
- The adductors (the inner thighs)

Some women have long, lean thigh muscles; in others, they're shorter and broader. 'Genetics is a primary factor in the size and shape of your thighs,' says Albohm. But so is use (or lack thereof).

The gluteals, quadriceps and hamstrings are the 'worker' muscles – the ones you use for running, jumping, climbing and lifting heavy objects. The adductors, in particular, suffer from neglect. Albohm compares flabby thighs to flabby upper arms. 'Women don't use their triceps – the underside of the upper arm – in any day-to-day activity, so they tend to get flabby,' she points out. 'The same thing happens to your inner thighs.' This also applies to your abductors, the outer thigh muscles. 'You use your quads, hamstrings and gluteals to move back and forth and up and down, but you don't move sideways very much,' explains Albohm. 'But work the inner and outer thigh muscles three days a week, and you'll see a difference.'

To tone and trim your hips, thighs and buttocks, 'you need a total-body workout with special emphasis on these muscle groups,' says Albohm, who designs workout programmes specifically for these areas. 'Your goal is to change the circumference of this area.' Combined with consistent aerobic exercise – and intelligent eating habits – the workouts that follow can help you reach your goal, she says. If you're just starting to exercise, go for the beginner exercises. If you are able to complete a designated programme with relative ease for three consecutive workout sessions, it's time to proceed to the next level.

You can expect to see some change in as little as 30 days, says Albohm.

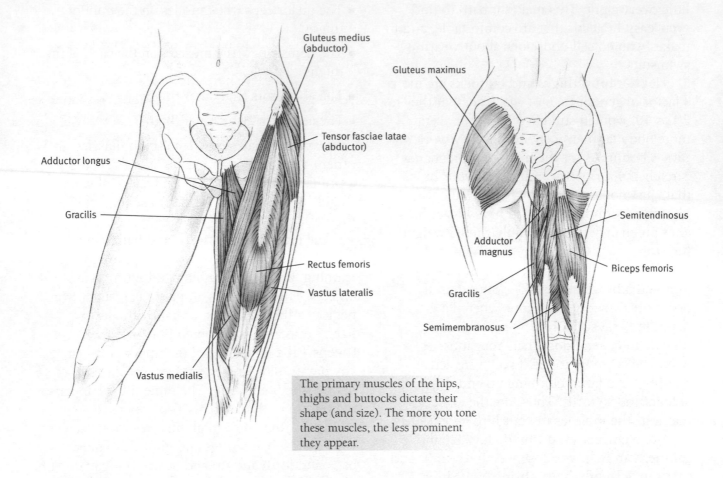

Gluteus medius
(abductor)

Gluteus maximus

Tensor fasciae latae
(abductor)

Adductor longus

Gracilis

Semitendinosus

Adductor
magnus

Rectus femoris

Biceps femoris

Vastus lateralis

Gracilis

Semimembranosus

Vastus medialis

The primary muscles of the hips,
thighs and buttocks dictate their
shape (and size). The more you tone
these muscles, the less prominent
they appear.

Working Smart

As with any exercise, there's a right and a wrong way to go about working your hips, thighs and buttocks.

Easy does it – at first. Start with the beginner programme until you get used to the movements. If you decide to add ankle weights to work your inner and outer thigh muscles, start with light weights and only a few reps. Don't exceed 5lb (2.3kg) – you completely change the leverage on your joints.

Do the exercise correctly to avoid injury. If you arch your back while you're doing the hip extension, for example, you could strain your back. And don't cheat – complete the full range of motion.

Make yourself comfortable. For some of the floor exercises, you'll need an exercise mat – or use a carpeted floor or large, folded towel.

But if you experience pain or discomfort when performing an exercise, stop and substitute another version. If pain persists, see your doctor.

Keep your movements tight and controlled. Don't swing your way through the exercise or let your muscles go slack.

Work your whole body. 'Despite what you may have heard, if it's strenuous enough – if you walk like you really mean it, for example – aerobic exercise can tone your muscles to some degree,' says Albohm. 'I do aerobics primarily for the cardiovascular effects, for example. But 20–30 per cent of my effort carries over to strengthen and tone my muscles.'

Step right up. Step aerobics is better for the hips, thighs and buttocks than regular aerobics, because it involves the quads, adductors, abductors and gluteals, says Albohm. Stair-climbing machines are good for the quads, hamstrings and gluteals – you work up and down in a straight line.

If you use a stair-climber, programme the machine to vary the resistance and height to give your muscles a thorough workout. (The same advice applies if you use an elliptical trainer or exercise bike.)

Measure your progress. It's a good idea to measure your hips, thighs and buttocks every month, not every week, says Albohm. 'Just be sure to measure at the same spot, in the same way, every time.' And don't be afraid that your hips, thighs and buttocks will get bigger when you follow this programme. 'Weight training will make muscles bigger only if it's done for that reason. There is a way to train to enlarge muscles – you have to use very, very heavy weights and very short ranges of motion with few repetitions. These exercises don't do that.'

Be consistent. 'To get the fastest results in the shortest period of time, do the exercises exactly as shown and make them part of your life,' says Albohm. 'Pay attention to the everyday versions of the exercises, so you'll be working these muscles every day, even when you don't have time to "work out".'

LEG EXTENSIONS

Muscles worked
Quadriceps (front thighs)

Performance hints

- Keep the working leg slightly bent throughout the motion.
- Maintain proper upper-body position throughout the exercise.
- Use your thigh muscles, not momentum, to lift your leg.

Intensity

Beginner: 3–10 reps with each leg, 3 days per week

Intermediate: 2 sets of 10 reps with each leg, 3 days per week

Experienced: 3 or 4 sets of 10 reps with each leg, 3 days per week. For additional resistance, add a 1- or 2lb (0.5- or 1.25kg) ankle weight to each leg.

Everyday version for quadriceps and gluteals

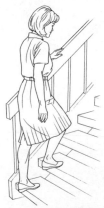

Use stairs rather than the lift. If there are many flights of stairs where you work, climb one flight for 3 weeks; increase the number of flights by 1 every 3 weeks. Or walk up and down the stairs in your home 3–5 extra times each day.

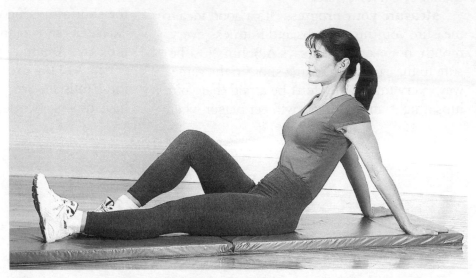

SUPPORTING YOUR TRUNK with your arms, sit on the floor with one leg extended, the knee slightly bent and foot flexed. Bend your opposite leg and place your foot flat on the floor.

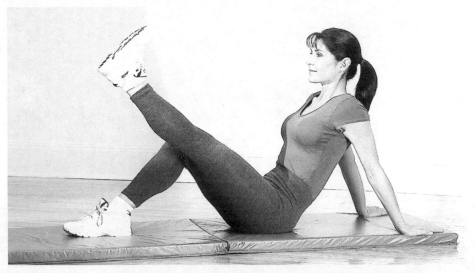

KEEPING YOUR KNEE slightly bent and your foot flexed, lift your leg in a slow and controlled movement until your knee reaches the height of the knee of your bent leg. Return to the starting position. Repeat with the other leg when the set is completed.

LUNGES

Muscles worked
Quadriceps (front thighs), gluteals (buttocks)

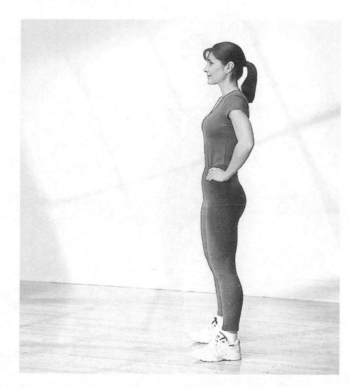

STAND WITH YOUR FEET about 6in (15cm) apart and your toes pointed straight ahead, in their natural position. For balance, rest your hands on your hips.

Performance hints

- Keep your torso from leaning forwards by looking straight ahead. Checking your position in a mirror may help.

- Do a full stretch with each lunge. Don't shorten the lunge as you do repetitions.

- Don't let your left knee extend beyond your toes.

- You should feel the stretch in your quadriceps.

Intensity

Beginner: 1 set of 3–10 reps with each leg, 3 days per week

Intermediate: 2 sets of 10 reps with each leg, 3 days per week

Experienced: 3 sets of 10 reps with each leg, 3 days per week, holding a 1- or 2lb/(0.5- or 1.25kg) dumbbell in each hand

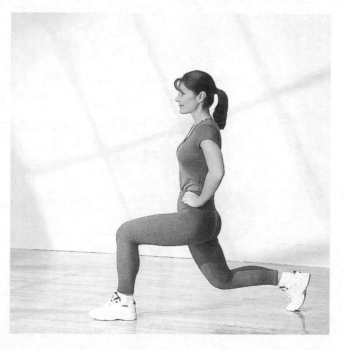

STEP FORWARD with your left foot as far as possible, bending your right knee as you do. In a controlled move, continue the lunge until your right knee almost touches the floor, and then slowly return to the starting position. Do one set, then repeat with the opposite leg.

SQUATS

Muscles worked
Quadriceps (front thighs), gluteals (buttocks)

Performance hints

- As you bend, keep your knees in direct line with your feet.
- Don't let your knees extend beyond your toes.
- Don't drop your buttocks lower than parallel to the floor.

Intensity

Beginner: 3–10 reps, 3 days per week

Intermediate: 2 sets of 10 reps, 3 days per week

Experienced: 3 sets of 10 reps, 3 days per week

Everyday version for quadriceps and gluteals

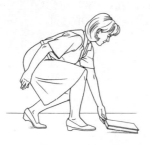

As you go about your daily activities, squat slightly to pick up or lift objects. (This is also safer than bending, because it protects the lower back from muscle injury.)

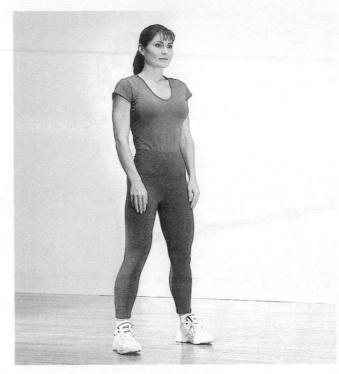

STAND WITH YOUR FEET shoulder-width apart. Tighten your abdomen and stand straight, looking directly ahead, focusing on a point so that your head and back are straight throughout the entire exercise.

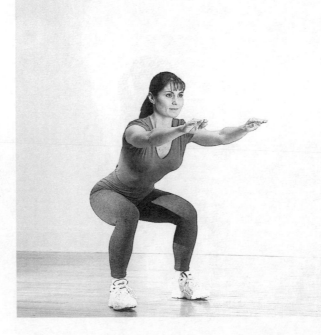

SLOWLY LOWER yourself into a squatting position by bending your legs at the knees. Descend enough for your thighs to be parallel to the ground. Return to the starting position. Repeat.

WALL SQUATS

Muscles worked
Quadriceps (front thighs)

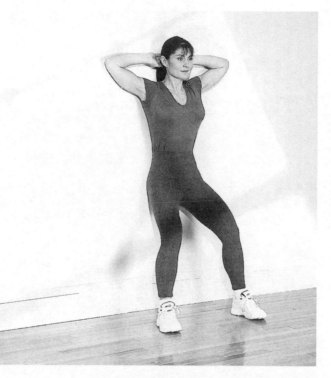

Performance hints

- Keep your trunk straight at all times.
- Don't bend your legs any lower than the point where your thighs are parallel to the floor.
- Use a slow, controlled motion.

Intensity

Beginner: 1 set of 3–10 reps, 3 days per week

Intermediate: 2 sets of 10 reps, 3 days per week

Experienced: 3 sets of 10 reps, 3 days per week

STAND AND LEAN BACK against a wall, feet shoulder-width apart, toes pointed slightly outwards. With your hands behind your head, your trunk straight and your shoulders back, 'walk' your feet forwards approximately 18 inches (45 cm) from the wall, or far enough so that your shins remain perpendicular to the floor.

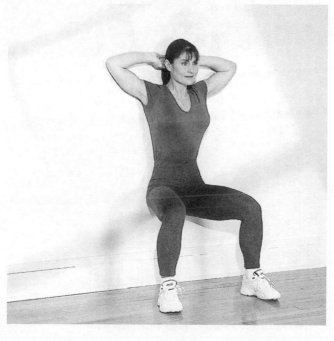

USING THE WALL to maintain balance, lower yourself in a slow, controlled movement until your thighs are parallel to the floor. Then return to the starting position and repeat.

LEG CURLS

Muscles worked
Hamstrings (backs of thighs)

Performance hints

- As you do this exercise concentrate on your hamstring muscles, tightening them as you raise your heel towards your buttocks.

- Keep the knee of the support leg slightly flexed.

- Use your hamstrings, not momentum, to perform this exercise.

Intensity

Beginner: 1 set of 3–10 reps, 3 days per week

Intermediate: 2 sets of 10 reps, 3 days per week

Experienced: 3 sets of 10 reps, 3 days per week. You can increase the effort by adding a 1lb (0.5kg) ankle weight to each leg.

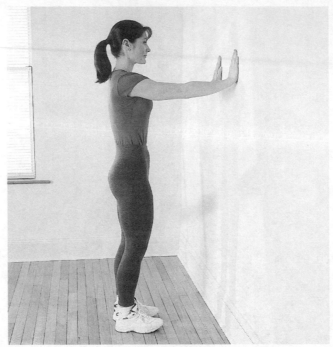

STAND FACING a wall with your hands on the wall for balance, and your feet approximately 12–15in (30–38cm) from the wall.

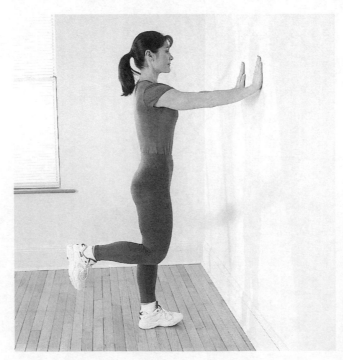

SLOWLY BEND one leg at the knee, raising the heel towards your buttocks in a slow, controlled movement until your lower leg is parallel to the floor. Do one set, then repeat with the opposite leg.

PRONE SINGLE-LEG RAISES

Muscles worked
Hamstrings (backs of thighs), gluteals (buttocks)

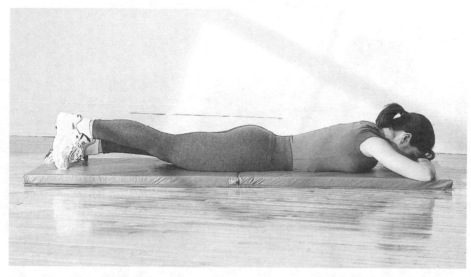

LIE FLAT on your stomach with your legs extended and your hands folded in front of you, with your forehead resting on your hands.

Performance hints

■ Don't raise your leg so high that you feel pain in your lower back.

■ Squeeze your buttocks as you raise your leg.

■ Keep the motion slow and controlled.

Intensity

Beginner: 1 set of 3–10 reps with each leg, 3 days per week

Intermediate: 2 sets of 10 reps with each leg, 3 days per week

Experienced: 3 sets of 10 reps with each leg, 3 days per week. To increase intensity further, you can add a 1- or 2lb (0.5- or 1.25kg) ankle weight to each ankle.

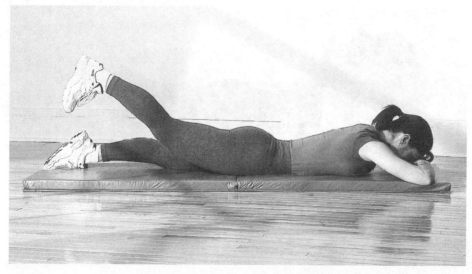

KEEPING YOUR LEG extended, your foot flexed and your knee slightly bent, raise one leg in a slow, controlled motion until you feel tightness in the muscles of your buttocks. Return to the starting position. Complete one set, then repeat with the other leg.

BACK LEG EXTENSIONS

Muscles worked
Hamstrings (backs of thighs), gluteals (buttocks)

Performance hints

- Keep your body stationary as you work each leg.
- Don't raise the extended leg so high that you feel pain in your lower back.
- Be sure to tighten your buttock muscles while performing this exercise.

Intensity

Beginner: 1 set of 3–10 reps with each leg, 3 days per week

Intermediate: 2 sets of 10 reps with each leg, 3 days per week

Experienced: 3 sets of 10 reps with each leg, 3 days per week. To increase intensity further, you can add a 1- or 2lb (0.5- or 1.25kg) ankle weight to each ankle.

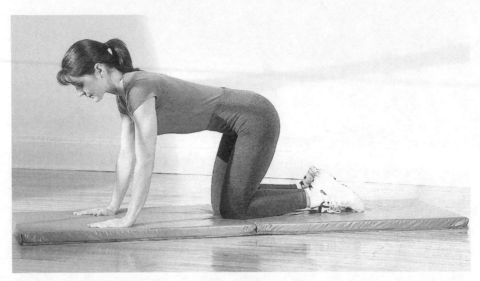

GET DOWN on all fours, with your arms fully extended, elbows locked, and your head and neck aligned with your spine.

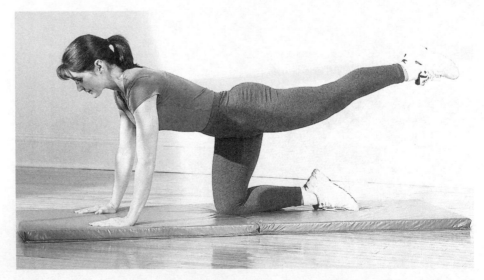

USING YOUR BUTTOCK muscles, extend and raise one leg until your thigh is parallel to the floor. Return to the starting position. Do one set, then repeat with the opposite leg.

BENT-LEG EXTENSIONS

Muscles worked
Hamstrings (backs of thighs), gluteals (buttocks)

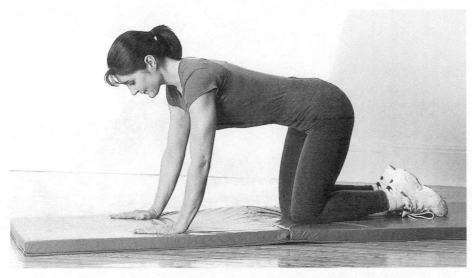

GET DOWN on all fours, with your arms fully extended, elbows locked, and your head and neck aligned with your spine.

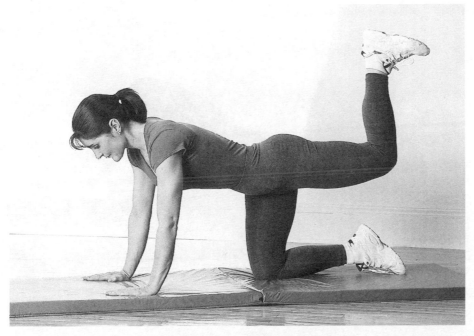

EXTEND ONE LEG, bent at a 90-degree angle, with your foot flexed, until your thigh is parallel to the ground. Return to the starting position. Do one set, then repeat with your other leg.

Performance hints

- Use one slow, continuous, controlled motion throughout the exercise.

- Don't extend the leg you're working higher than parallel to the floor.

- Use your buttock muscles, not momentum, to raise your leg.

Intensity

Beginner: 1 set of 3–10 reps with each leg, 3 days per week

Intermediate: 2 sets of 10 reps with each leg, 3 days per week

Experienced: 3 sets of 10 reps with each leg, 3 days per week. You can increase resistance by adding a 1- or 2lb (0.5- or 1.25kg) ankle weight to each leg.

Everyday version for gluteals, hamstrings and outer thighs

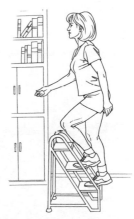

Spend 3–5 minutes climbing and descending a stepladder, for 30 seconds at a time, with a 15-second rest between 30-second periods.

PELVIC LIFTS

Muscles worked

Hamstrings (backs of thighs), gluteals (buttocks)

Performance hints

- Raise your hips only until your back is straight. Don't arch your back.
- Keep your buttock muscles contracted at all times.
- Use a slow, controlled motion.

Intensity

Beginner: 1 set of 10 reps, 3 days per week

Intermediate: 2 sets of 10 reps, 3 days per week

Experienced: 3 sets of 10 reps, 3 days per week

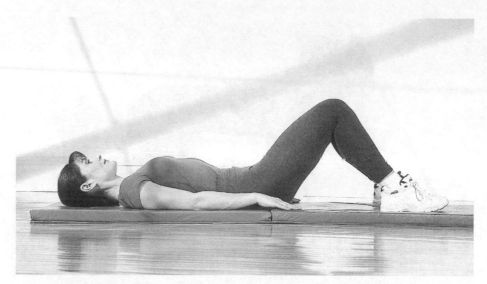

LIE ON YOUR BACK with your knees bent and your feet flat on the floor, with your hands at your sides, palms down.

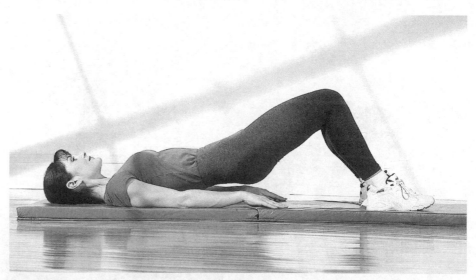

LIFT YOUR PELVIS towards the ceiling, squeezing your buttocks, until your back is straight. Repeat.

BENT-KNEE CROSSOVERS

Muscles worked
Gluteals (buttocks), hamstrings (backs of thighs), abductors (outer thighs)

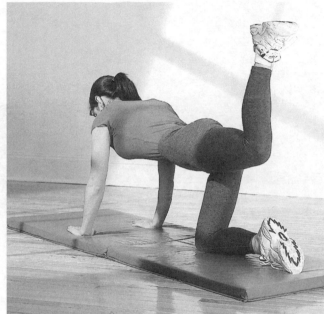

GET DOWN on all fours with your back flat, then bend and raise one leg.

Performance hints

- Keep your thigh parallel to the floor at the top of the motion.
- To initiate the exercise, move your foot towards the ceiling.
- Use one slow, controlled movement throughout the exercise.

Intensity

Beginner: 1 set of 3–10 reps with each leg, 3 days per week

Intermediate: 2 sets of 10 reps with each leg, 3 days per week

Experienced: 3 sets of 10 reps with each leg, 3 days per week. You can increase the intensity by adding a 1lb (0.5kg) ankle weight to each leg.

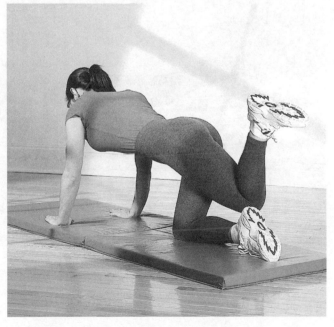

KEEPING THE RAISED LEG bent at a 90-degree angle throughout the exercise, lift your leg up and back, crossing over the calf of the non-working leg. Keep your buttocks tight at all times. Return to the starting position. Do one set, then repeat with the other leg.

SIDE-LYING STRAIGHT-LEG RAISES

Muscles worked
Gluteals (buttocks), abductors (outer thighs)

Performance hints

- Keep your upper leg rotated downwards.
- Keep your upper body stable.
- Use a slow, controlled motion.

Intensity

Beginner: 1 set of 3–10 reps with each leg, 3 days per week

Intermediate: 2 sets of 10 reps with each leg, 3 days per week

Experienced: 3 sets of 10 reps with each leg, 3 days per week. You can increase resistance by adding a 1- or 2lb (0.5- or 1.25kg) ankle weight to each leg.

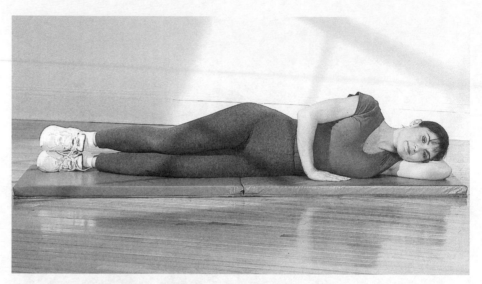

LIE ON YOUR SIDE with your legs together, supporting your head with one arm and balancing yourself with the other.

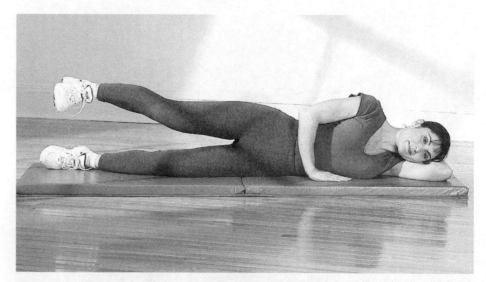

KEEPING YOUR upper leg rotated in (toe pointing down) and your foot flexed, raise the top leg in a slow, controlled motion approximately 10–12in (20–30cm) off the floor without moving your torso. Return to the starting position. Do one set, then repeat with the opposite leg.

STANDING ABDUCTIONS

Muscles worked
Gluteals (buttocks), abductors (outer thighs)

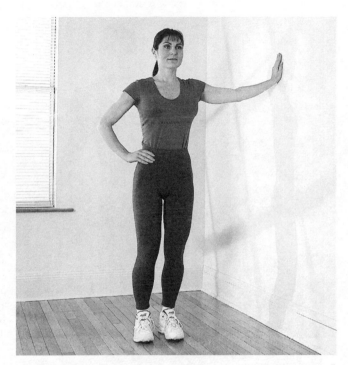

HOLDING ON to a wall for balance, stand with your knees slightly bent.

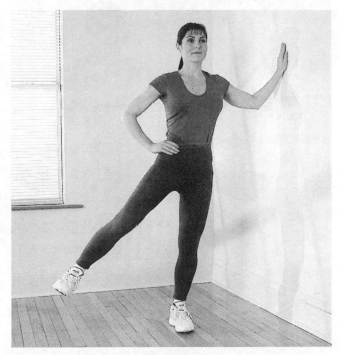

KEEPING YOUR KNEE slightly bent, lift the working leg to the side. Your foot should be flexed. Lift as far as you can without moving your upper torso. Return to the starting position. Do one set, then repeat with the opposite leg.

Performance hints

- Use the muscles of your outer thigh and hip to lift your leg.
- Keep the stationary leg slightly flexed.
- Lift the leg in a slow, controlled movement.
- Don't twist your shoulders and chest.

Intensity

Beginner: 1 set of 3–10 reps with each leg, 3 days per week

Intermediate: 2 sets of 10 reps with each leg, 3 days per week

Experienced: 3 sets of 10 reps with each leg, 3 days per week. You can increase resistance by adding a 1- or 2lb (0.5- or 1.25kg) ankle weight to each leg.

Everyday version for gluteals and abductors

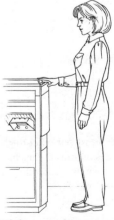

While standing, contract your buttocks, hold for 6–8 seconds, and then release. Do for 1–3 minutes, 2–3 times per day.

141

SEATED ABDUCTIONS

Muscles worked
Abductors (outer thighs)

Performance hints

- Keep your knee slightly flexed and your foot flexed throughout the motion.

- Don't move your upper body.

Intensity

Beginner: 1 set of 3–10 reps with each leg, 3 days per week

Intermediate: 2 sets of 10 reps with each leg, 3 days per week

Experienced: 3 sets of 10 reps with each leg, 3 days per week. You can increase resistance by adding a 1- or 2lb (0.5- or 1.25kg) ankle weight to each leg.

Everyday version for abductors

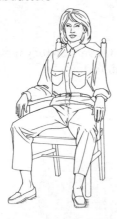

While seated, press your outer thighs against the sides or arms of the chair; hold for 6–8 seconds. Repeat for 1–3 minutes, 3 times per day.

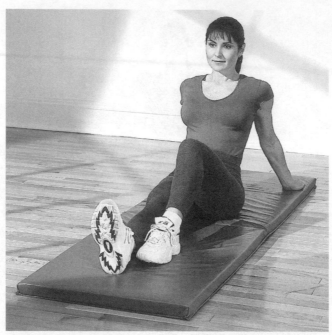

WHILE SUPPORTING your upper body with your arms and with your elbows slightly bent, sit on the floor with one leg extended and the knee slightly bent and foot flexed.

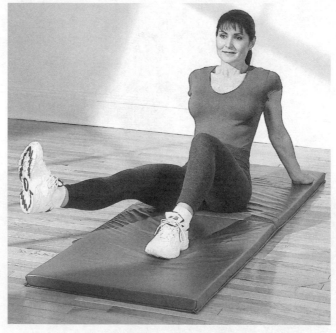

KEEPING YOUR knee slightly bent and your foot flexed, move the working leg to the side as far as you can, without moving your torso. Return to the starting position. Do one set, then repeat with the other leg.

SIDE-LYING BENT-LEG RAISES

Muscles worked
Abductors (outer thighs)

Performance hints

- Keep the knee of your upper leg bent and your foot flexed throughout the motion.
- Keep your upper body still throughout the exercise.

Intensity

Beginner: 1 set of 3–10 reps with each leg, 3 days per week

Intermediate: 2 sets of 10 reps with each leg, 3 days per week

Experienced: 3 sets of 10 reps with each leg, 3 days per week. You can increase resistance by adding a 1- or 2lb (0.5- or 1.25kg) ankle weight to each leg.

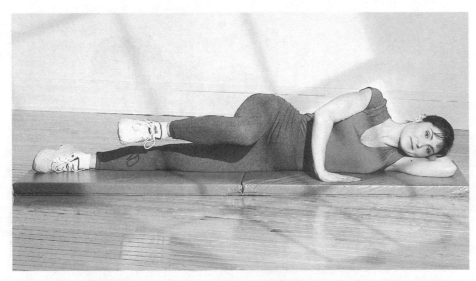

LIE ON YOUR SIDE with your bottom leg straight and your top leg perpendicular to your body, with the knee bent at 90 degrees. Support your head with your bottom arm and stabilise your body by placing the palm of the other hand down in front of your chest.

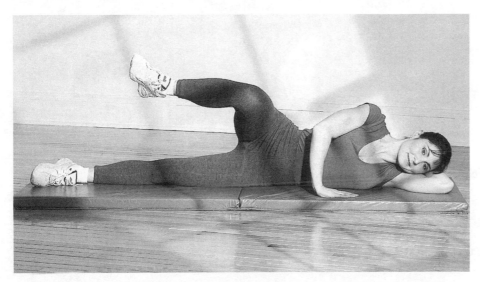

KEEPING YOUR TOP LEG perpendicular to your body, raise it up in a slow and controlled motion as high as you can without twisting your torso or compromising your foot position. Return to the starting position and repeat with your other leg when the set is complete.

FIRE HYDRANTS

Muscles worked
Abductors (outer thighs), adductors (inner thighs), gluteals (buttocks)

Performance hints
- To keep your back straight and your spine properly aligned, hold your head straight (not raised or lowered).
- Perform this exercise in a slow, controlled, continuous motion.

Intensity
Beginner: 1 set of 3–10 reps with each leg, 3 days per week

Intermediate: 2 sets of 10 reps with each leg, 3 days per week

Experienced: 3 sets of 10 reps with each leg, 3 days per week

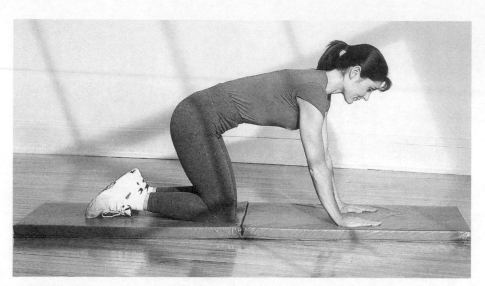

GET DOWN ON ALL FOURS, with your arms extended, your elbows locked and your back parallel to the floor.

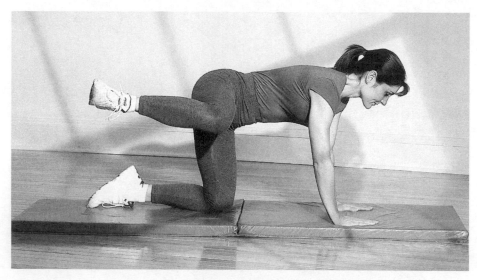

LIFT ONE LEG to the side at a 90-degree angle until it is parallel to the floor. Return to the starting position. Do one set, then repeat with the opposite leg.

INNER LEG RAISES

Muscles worked
Adductors (inner thighs)

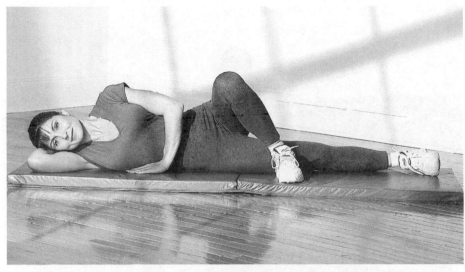

LIE ON YOUR SIDE, supporting your head with your arm and your upper body with your opposite hand. Bend your top leg and place it in front of your other leg so your foot is flat on the floor and your bottom leg is straight with the knee slightly bent and the foot flexed.

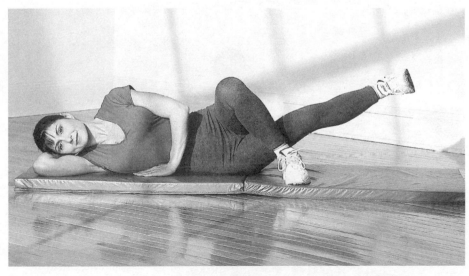

RAISE YOUR BOTTOM LEG as high as possible without moving the rest of your body. Return to the starting position without touching your foot to the floor. Do one set, then repeat with your other leg.

Performance hints

- Keep your upper body still.
- Keep your inner thigh facing the ceiling.
- Perform the movement in a slow, controlled manner.

Intensity

Beginner: 1 set of 3–10 reps with each leg, 3 days per week

Intermediate: 2 sets of 10 reps with each leg, 3 days per week

Experienced: 3 sets of 10 reps with each leg, 3 days per week. You can increase resistance by adding a 1- or 2lb (0.5- or 1.25kg) ankle weight to each leg.

Everyday version for adductors

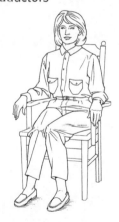

While seated, contract your inner thigh muscles by pushing your knees together; hold for 6–8 seconds. Release. Do for 1–3 minutes, 3 times per day.

SEATED INNER LEG RAISES

Muscles worked
Adductors (inner thighs)

Performance hints

- Keep the leg you're working 1in (2.5cm) above the floor at all times.
- Keep your upper torso straight and square to the rest of your body.
- Perform the movement in a slow, controlled motion.

Intensity

Beginner: 1 set of 3–10 reps with each leg, 3 days per week

Intermediate: 2 sets of 10 reps with each leg, 3 days per week

Experienced: 3 sets of 10 reps with each leg, 3 days per week. You can increase resistance by adding a 1- or 2lb (0.5- or 1.25kg) ankle weight to each leg.

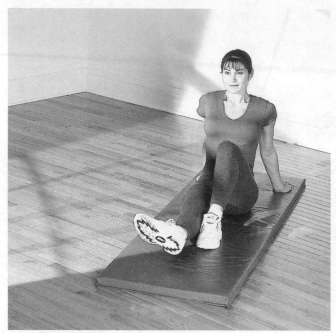

SIT WITH ONE LEG bent and the foot flat on the floor, leaning back and supporting yourself. Extend the other leg, bending your knee slightly, flexing your foot and rotating your hip (toes pointed out).

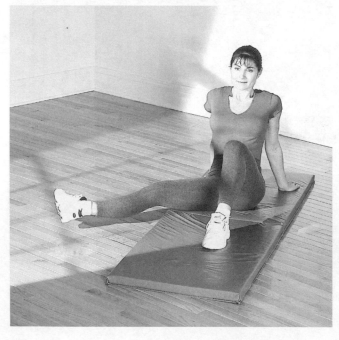

MOVE THE WORKING LEG outwards as far as you can without losing your balance. Return to the starting position without touching your foot to the floor. Do one set, then repeat with your other leg.

BUTTERFLY LEG RAISES

Muscles worked
Adductors (inner thighs)

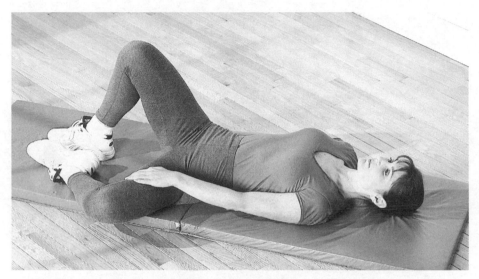

LIE ON YOUR BACK with one leg bent and the foot flat on the floor, and the other leg bent and lowered to the side. The sole of the foot of the lowered leg should face the side of the other foot.

Performance hints

- Keep both legs bent throughout the motion.
- Using your hand, provide as much resistance as needed to make the exercise challenging.
- Keep your lower back pressed to the floor.

Intensity

Beginner: 1 set of 3–10 reps with each leg, 3 days per week

Intermediate: 2 sets of 10 reps with each leg, 3 days per week

Experienced: 3 sets of 10 reps with each leg, 3 days per week

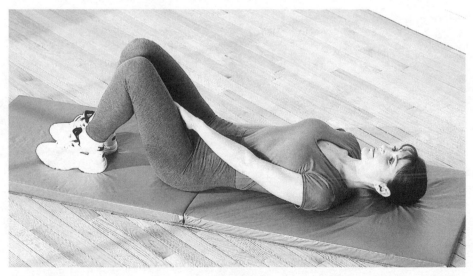

KEEPING YOUR LEGS BENT, raise the lowered knee towards the opposite knee, pressing against the inner thigh with your hands, for resistance. Return to the starting position. Do one set, then repeat with the other leg.

SINGLE-LEG PELVIC LIFTS

Muscles worked
Gluteals (buttocks) and adductors (inner thighs)

Performance hints

- Raise your pelvis until your back is straight, but no higher (not arched).
- Keep your buttock muscles contracted at all times.
- Perform this move in a slow, controlled manner.

Intensity

Beginner: 1 set of 10 reps, 3 days per week

Intermediate: 2 sets of 10 reps, 3 days per week

Experienced: 3 sets of 10 reps, 3 days per week. You can increase the intensity by straightening your leg instead of resting it on the other knee.

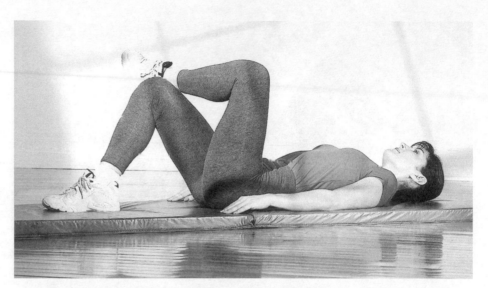

LIE ON YOUR BACK with one knee bent and the foot flat on the floor, with your hands at your sides. Cross the opposite leg over the bent leg, with your ankle resting just above the knee.

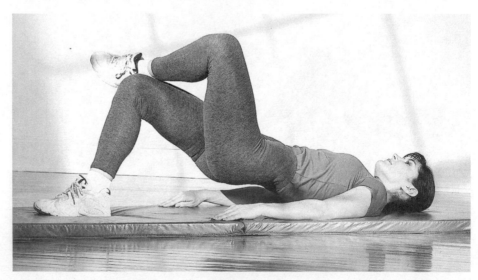

RAISE YOUR PELVIS towards the ceiling, squeezing the muscles in your buttocks as you lift. Return to the starting position. Do one set, then repeat with the other leg.

SCISSORS

Muscles worked
Adductors (inner thighs), abductors (outer thighs)

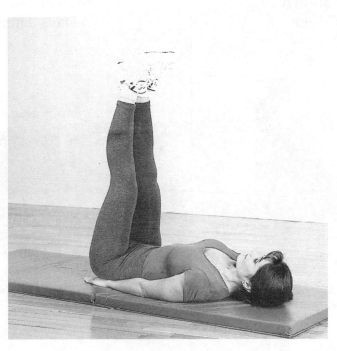

LIE ON YOUR BACK with your head resting on the floor. Place your palms flat on the floor under your buttocks and raise your legs, with your knees slightly bent, almost perpendicular to the floor. Your feet should be slightly flexed with your toes pointed slightly outwards.

Performance hints

- Use your inner and outer thigh muscles, not momentum, to perform the exercise.
- Keep your back flat on the floor.
- As you perform the exercise, maintain muscle tension in your inner and outer thighs.

Intensity

Beginner: 1 set of 10 reps, 3 days per week

Intermediate: 2 sets of 10 reps, 3 days per week

Experienced: 3 sets of 10 reps, 3 days per week. Use rubber tubing attached at your ankles or lower-leg area to increase the intensity.

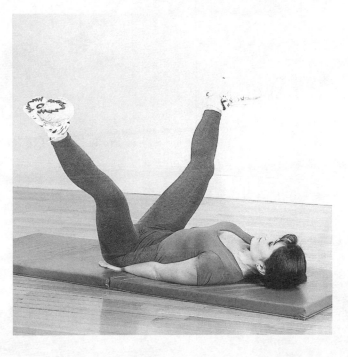

USING A SLOW, controlled movement, spread your legs as far apart as possible. Return to the starting position. Repeat.

149

30-Day Beginner Programme

Week 1

Do Exercises Shown
3 Days This Week

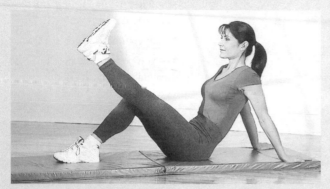

Leg Extensions (page 130)

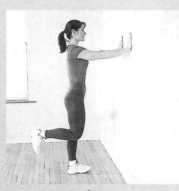

Leg Curls (page 134)

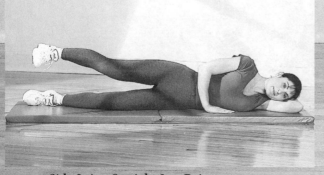

Side-Lying Straight-Leg Raises (page 140)

Week 2

Do Exercises Shown
3 Days This Week

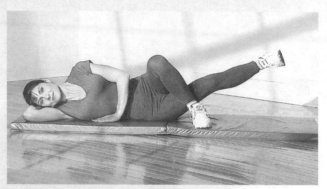

Inner Leg Raises (page 145)

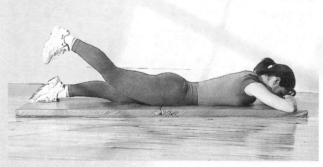

Prone Single-Leg Raises (page 135)

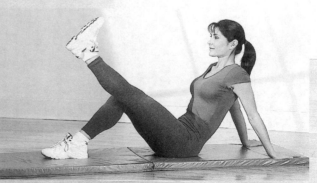

Leg Extensions (page 130)

Week 3

Do Exercises Shown
3 Days This Week

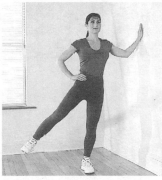

Standing Abductions (page 141)

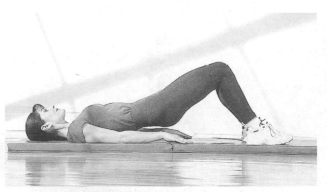

Pelvic Lifts (page 138)

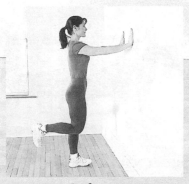

Leg Curls (page 134)

Week 4

Do Exercises Shown
3 Days This Week

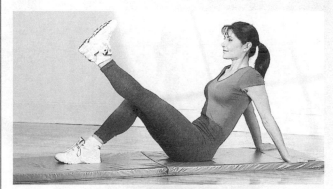

Leg Extensions (page 130)

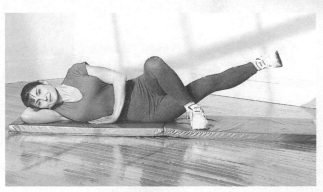

Inner Leg Raises (page 145)

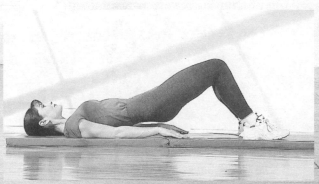

Pelvic Lifts (page 138)

30-Day Intermediate Programme

Week 1

Do Exercises Shown
3 Days This Week

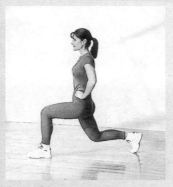

Lunges (page 131)

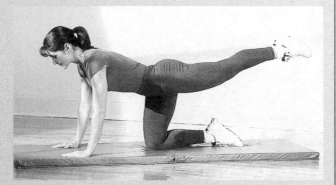

Back Leg Extensions (page 136)

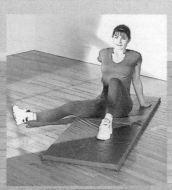

Seated Inner Leg Raises (page 146)

Week 2

Do Exercises Shown
3 Days This Week

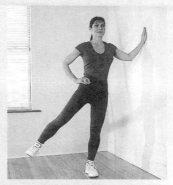

Standing Abductions (page 141)

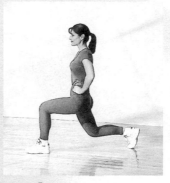

Lunges (page 131)

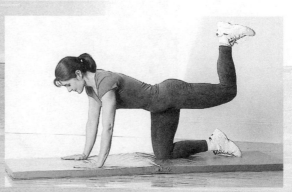

Bent-Leg Extensions (page 137)

Week 3

Do Exercises Shown
3 Days This Week

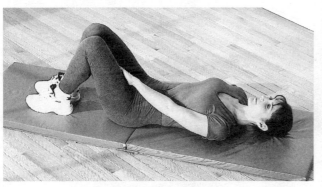

Butterfly Leg Raises (page 147)

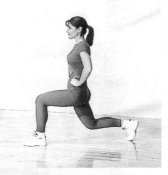

Lunges (page 131)

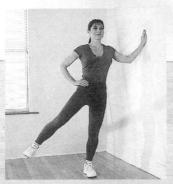

Standing Abductions (page 141)

Week 4

Do Exercises Shown
3 Days This Week

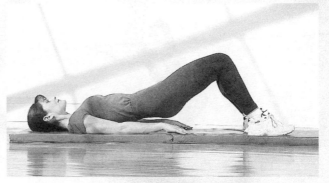

Pelvic Lifts (page 138)

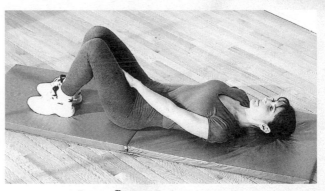

Butterfly Leg Raises (page 147)

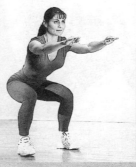

Squats (page 132)

30-Day Experienced Programme

Week 1

Do Exercises Shown
3 Days This Week

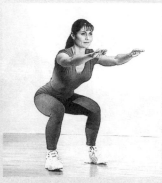

Squats (page 132)

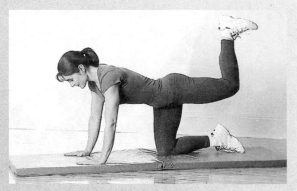

Bent-Leg Extensions (page 137)

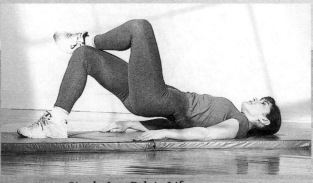

Single-Leg Pelvic Lifts (page 148)

Week 2

Do Exercises Shown
3 Days This Week

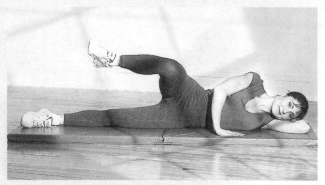

Side-Lying Bent-Leg Raises (page 140)

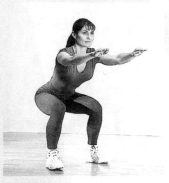

Squats (page 132)

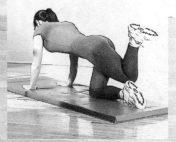

Bent-Knee Crossovers (page 139)

Week 3

Do Exercises Shown
3 Days This Week

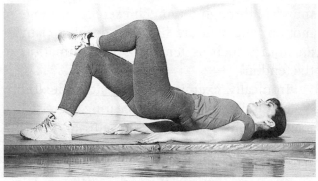

Single-Leg Pelvic Lifts (page 148)

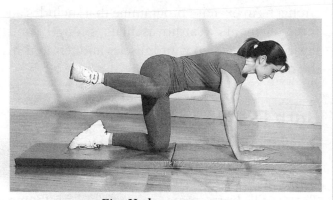

Fire Hydrants (page 144)

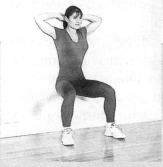

Wall Squats (page 133)

Week 4

Do Exercises Shown
3 Days This Week

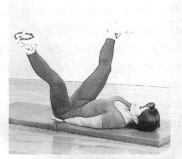

Scissors (page 149)

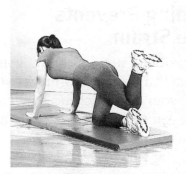

Bent-Knee Crossovers (page 139)

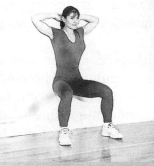

Wall Squats (page 133)

Chapter 10

Stretch into Shape

Stretching keeps your muscles flexible, helping to prepare them for exercise and recover from the effort afterwards. Skip the stretches, and you won't get the benefits you should from aerobic exercise and resistance training.

'Stretching helps you move freely during aerobic exercise, it enables your muscles to build more strength during weight training, and it helps keep muscles long and lean,' says sports trainer Sharon Willett.

Contrary to what you may have heard in the past, experts agree that before stretching you should warm up your muscles, to avoid tearing 'cold' or stiff muscles.

Stretching Prevents Muscle Strain

Lack of flexibility not only slows your progress but can lead to injury. And unless you've been athletic all your life, the chances are you're not as flexible as you need to be to get the most out of your body-toning workouts.

When you were a baby, you were so flexible that you could probably put your big toe in your mouth. When you were a teenager, you could slither under a limbo bar. But as we age, both our muscles and tendons lose their flexibility. If the only exercise we get is flipping through the TV listings, our muscles flex even less, getting stiffer over the years.

'Our habits and daily activities can also cause our muscles and tendons to shorten,' says Willett. Even your shoes can inhibit your flexibility. For example, wearing high heels shortens the hamstrings and calves. This won't be a problem when you're sitting still, but if you try to do a leg curl or squat, the shortened muscles won't do the

job willingly. Try to push a shortened muscle or tendon (the strands of tissue that attach bones to muscles) through too much exercise or range of motion, and you are likely to develop pain or an injury, such as tendinitis (inflammation of the tendon).

Ironically, exercise too can affect flexibility. 'Weight training and weight-bearing exercise like jogging contract muscles again and again, shortening the muscles and tendons involved,' says Willett. 'So you have to stretch out your muscles again after you use them. If you do so, not only will your muscles and tendons retain their elasticity but they'll be able to get even stronger. An exercise programme that includes all three elements (cardiovascular, strength and flexibility) will keep your muscles and tendons in the best shape possible.'

Burn Fat While You Stretch

In addition to keeping you flexible, stretching burns calories.

'Stretching isn't aerobic,' concedes Willett. 'But you'll burn more calories by stretching than you will by sitting and doing nothing.' For a 10½ stone (67-kilo) woman, 30 minutes of stretching burns 60–100 calories – about the same as very gentle yoga – compared to 22 calories for sitting still.

As an added incentive you'll find that stretching is extremely relaxing, especially after a workout. 'Stretching will slowly lower your heart rate after an activity,' says Willett. 'That has a calming effect on most people. Also, the deep breathing and stillness required for stretching are really helpful for releasing tension both in the muscles and in the mind.'

The Right Way to Stretch

Experts recommend that you stretch all your muscle groups, rather than just targetting your particular trouble spot. All your muscles and tendons work together, so if you ignore one stretch you won't get maximum benefit from the others.

As for how to stretch, it should come fairly naturally. We raise our arms when we get out of bed; we wiggle our backs if we feel a muscle ache. All of these motions are really stretches. It's easy. Still, for maximum effectiveness you need to keep a few rules in mind when you stretch, says Willett.

Warm your muscles. Stretching is not a warm-up. Spend at least five minutes doing some form of light aerobic exercise, such as walking, climbing stairs or cleaning the house. Work hard enough to feel warm and sweat slightly. If you stretch after your workout, your muscles will be warm and supple.

Don't bounce. Pushing your muscles in short, jerky movements tears the fibres. Instead, slowly and evenly move into the stretch until you feel resistance, then back off a little and hold that position.

Hold each stretch for 20 seconds. 'Stretches held for at least 20 seconds increase flexibility the most,' says Willett. And don't hold your breath. Instead, take two or three deep breaths as you hold the stretch.

Do each stretch two, three or four times. The real benefits come in increments, with each subsequent stretch.

When (and How Often) to Stretch

Stretching doesn't take much time – as little as 10 minutes should do it. And it's easy to fit into a busy workout schedule – all you need is an exercise mat or an improvised one. As for when to stretch, you have a number of options.

- If you've just begun your exercise programme, it's best to stretch each muscle group immediately after an activity in which you've used those muscles, says Willett. So if you're doing squats to tone your butt, for example, stretch the gluteus muscles immediately after the exercise. And if you're working out every day, that means you'll stretch every day.

- If you're comfortable with your routine and never ache afterwards, says Willett, feel free to do all of your stretches at the end of your workout.

- If it's convenient, you can also stretch without doing other exercise (except warming up). You'll benefit from two half-hour sessions a week even on days when you don't exercise.

'You can even stretch while you watch TV,' says Willett. 'There's no reason to be formal about it.'

PRESS-UPS

Muscles stretched
Upper and lower abs

Easier version: prop-up

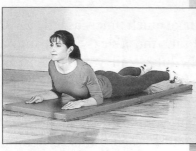

If you're unable to do the regular version because of wrist, arm or lower back pain, prop yourself up on your forearms and raise your chest up while keeping your hips on the floor.

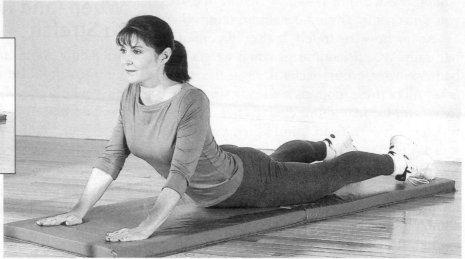

LIE ON YOUR STOMACH with your hands on the floor, directly under your shoulders. Raise your upper body as far as you can by straightening your elbows and arching your back, keeping your hips in contact with the floor. Keep your chest upright so your shoulders are not hunched up by your ears. You should feel the stretch along the front of your body. You can lift your chin, but don't drop your head back. Hold for 20–30 seconds. Repeat four times.

KNEE SQUEEZES

Muscles stretched
Upper, middle and lower back muscles

Easier version:
Single-knee squeeze

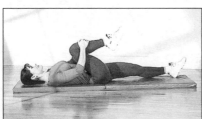

If you're unable to work both knees at the same time, start by bringing one knee up to your chest and holding the stretch for 20–30 seconds. Relax and repeat with the opposite knee. Also, you don't have to bring your head up off the floor if it puts too much strain on your neck.

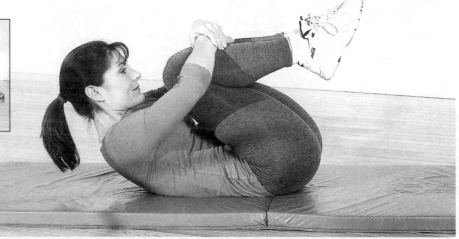

LIE ON YOUR BACK with your legs outstretched. Bend both knees and hold. Bring them towards your chest until you feel a stretch. Tuck your chin in and slowly bring your head up to meet your knees. Stay relaxed. Hold for 20–30 seconds. Repeat four times.

SPINAL TWISTS

Muscles stretched
Middle and lower back muscles

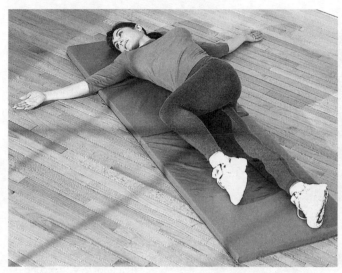

LIE ON YOUR BACK with your arms out to each side (perpendicular to your body). Keeping your shoulders flat on the floor, bend your left knee up towards your chest and slowly bring the bent leg across your body. Turn your head to look at your right hand until you feel a stretch. Hold for 20–30 seconds, then repeat on the other side. Do four stretches on each side.

FIGURE FOUR STRETCHES

Muscles stretched
Gluteus maximus (buttocks)

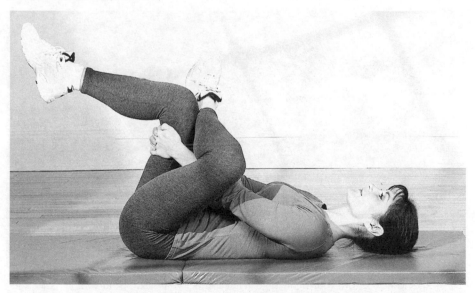

LIE ON YOUR BACK with both knees bent. Cross your left foot over your right knee. Place your hands behind your right knee and slowly bring your knee towards your chest. You should feel the stretch in your left buttock area. Hold for 20–30 seconds, then repeat on the opposite side. Stretch each side four times.

HIP FLEXOR STRETCHES

Muscles stretched
Muscles in front of the hips and thighs

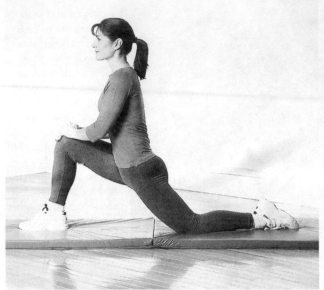

BEGIN BY KNEELING on the floor. Bring your right knee in front of you and place your foot flat on the floor. Your left knee should be resting on the floor. Slowly lean forward to extend your left leg back, keeping your shin and knee on the floor. You should feel a stretch in the front of your right hip and thigh. Make sure your right knee isn't extending further than your toes. (If it is, move your right leg farther back.) Hold this stretch for 20–30 seconds, then switch sides. Repeat four times.

HIP/QUAD STRETCHES

Muscle stretched
Iliotibial band (outside of legs from hips to knees) and quadriceps

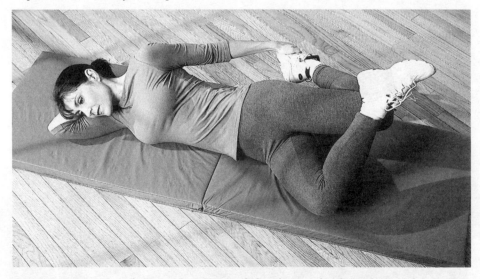

LIE ON YOUR RIGHT SIDE with your right arm extended under your head. Bend your left knee and use your left hand to pull your heel up towards your buttock. Take your right foot and place it on top of your left knee. Apply a downward pressure with your right foot, pushing your left knee towards the floor. Hold for 20–30 seconds and then repeat on the opposite side. Repeat the stretch four times on each side.

INNER THIGH AND GROIN STRETCHES

Muscles stretched
Inner thighs and groin

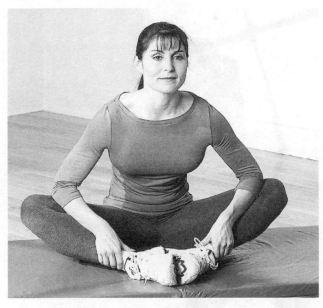

SIT ON THE FLOOR with your back straight. Place the heels of your feet together and drop your knees out to your sides. Clasp your hands around your ankles. Using your forearms, slowly press your knees towards the floor until you feel a stretch. Don't force your knees to the floor. Hold for 20–30 seconds. Repeat four times.

HAMSTRING STRETCHES

Muscles stretched
Backs of thighs

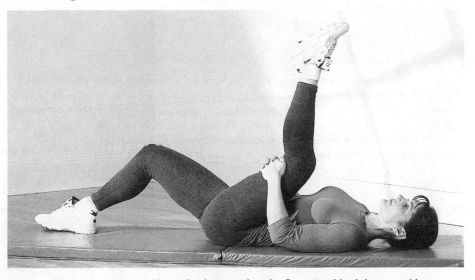

LIE ON YOUR BACK, keeping your lower back pressed to the floor. Bend both knees and keep your feet flat on the floor. Bring your hands to the back of your left thigh and slowly straighten and raise your left leg. Gently pull your leg in towards your torso until you feel a stretch in the back of your leg. Hold for 20–30 seconds, then repeat with the other leg. Repeat four times with each leg. As this stretch becomes easier, keep the resting leg straight out in front of you instead of bent, for more of a stretch.

CALF STRETCHES

Muscles stretched

Gastrocnemius and soleus (backs and sides of calves) and Achilles tendon

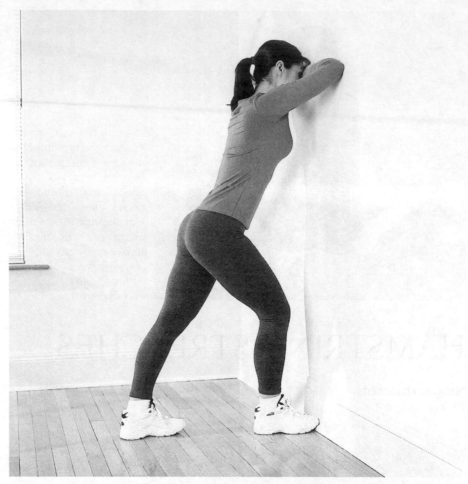

STAND WITH YOUR FOREARMS against a wall and your right leg out in front of you with the knee bent. Your knees shouldn't extend past your toes. Keep your left leg straight and your foot flat on the floor. Slowly lean forwards on your right leg until you feel a stretch in the back of your calf. Hold for 20–30 seconds. This will stretch the upper part of the calf. Then slightly bend your left knee and repeat to stretch the lower part of the calf. Hold each stretch for 20–30 seconds, then switch sides. Repeat four times with each leg.

PART FOUR

Aerobics for Overall Slimness

Chapter 11

Twenty-five Ways to Work Off Fat and Calories

Thanks to a daily aerobic workout that consisted only of walking (coupled with weight training), Barbara lost 23in (58cm), mostly from her waist, abdomen and hips.

'I am quite overweight and have a long way to go,' says Barbara, 51, a nursing assistant. 'But I can't believe I started to see changes in just one month! Sometimes I just can't find time to walk. But on those days I spend one to two hours at a time weeding my garden.'

Working out aerobically doesn't mean you have to run or join a class to lose weight and shape up – unless you want to. Everyday activities like walking and gardening burn fat and calories just like more strenuous workouts and can help women just like you flatten their abs, trim their thighs and slim their butts.

How It Works

Aerobic exercise works this way: your exertion demands an increased flow of oxygen to supply energy. When you breathe in, the oxygen pours from your lungs into your bloodstream. Your heart then pumps it to your muscles. There, the oxygen is used to break down carbohydrate, fat and protein into the energy that your muscles need to function.

Aerobic activities are big calorie burners, and – along with a diet that limits fat and calories – they go a long way towards melting away fat. That's because causing your heart to pump at a faster, sustained rate will increase your metabolism during the exercise, burning more calories, and it may eventually increase your metabolic rate, the rate at which you burn calories as you go about your daily business. Metabolic changes, in turn, improve your body's ability to burn fat and make your muscles better able to use oxygen for this purpose. As your level of aerobic fitness increases, your heart, lungs and muscles become more efficient, so you can do more without getting tired.

Once you become more physically active, people may start noticing that you look leaner and more muscular. Most aerobic activity doesn't build muscle, but your muscles will look more toned and you'll lose fat. For that reason, your clothes will fit better even before you see your weight change on the scales.

Looking good isn't the only benefit: you'll feel good, too. Evidence shows that participating in aerobic exercise can help reduce symptoms of depression and anxiety and make you feel better emotionally. A study conducted by the department of human performance and health promotion at the University of New Orleans, for example, found that 36 women and six men who enrolled in step aerobics classes of varying intensity felt less tense, depressed, fatigued and angry after the more intense workouts than they did after the less intense workouts.

Some experts say that exercise elevates your mood simply by freeing your mind from everyday concerns. It may just be that you're enjoying yourself. Given that many women tend to overeat when they're tired, bored, tense or angry, the psychological benefits of aerobic exercise can play a part in your success.

No one is exactly sure why exercise elevates mood. Other authorities say that during and after exercise your brain releases endorphins, chemical substances associated with pleasure. You've probably heard athletes or others refer to this as an endorphin high. But everyday exercisers like you can enjoy the same uplifting effect.

How Hard Do You Have to Work?

To reap the health benefits of aerobic exercise, you need to work at moderate intensity to raise your heart rate for at least 30 minutes a day three to five times a week.

If you're aiming to lose weight, you need to exercise aerobically at moderate intensity for 30–60 minutes most days of the week. Thirty minutes is the point at which fat starts to be used as the primary energy source.

How do you know what's moderate intensity? One way is to calculate your target heart rate. To do this, subtract your age from 220. This tells you your approximate maximum heart rate. You don't want to work at your maximum (nor should you). Instead, you need to calculate your target heart rate zone – a range, depending on your fitness level. To do that, multiply your maximum rate by 0.6 if you want to exercise at 60 per cent of your maximum (low intensity), which is good for beginners, 0.7 for 70 per cent of your maximum (moderate intensity) or 0.8 for 80 per cent (high intensity). Once you're in pretty good shape, you can work up to 90 per cent.

To calculate her target heart rate zone, for example, Sarah, the 52-year-old described in earlier chapters, would subtract 52 from 220 to arrive at her maximum heart rate of 168. To work out at 70 per cent of this maximum rate she would multiply 168 by 0.7 to arrive at a target heart rate of 118.

You can make sure your heart rate falls within your target range while you exercise by placing two or three fingers – but not your thumb, which has its own pulse – lightly in the inside of your opposite wrist below the base of your thumb. Count the beats for one minute to get the pulse rate, which is the beat of the heart as felt through the walls of the arteries, or count for 15 seconds and multiply by four.

If you have no patience with numbers, there are simpler ways to tell if you're exercising hard enough You're doing fine if you're breathing hard, but not so hard that you can't carry on a conversation. Or if you've broken into a sweat. Or if you simply *feel* like you're working.

Alternatively, ask yourself how much longer you can carry on the activity. It should take enough out of you that you wouldn't be able to continue for hours, but you shouldn't be working so hard that you need to stop right away.

As you continue to get in shape, what used to be strenuous will become easier, so you must add to the duration, intensity or frequency of the exercise, or start doing a different, more challenging activity. For each of the aerobic activities described in the pages that follow, experts have prescribed beginner, intermediate and experienced levels to help you get started and progress. These levels are not just for safety; they have a built-in success ratio. Allow yourself 20–30 minutes a day, and make your workout part of your daily routine.

Work Hard (but Not Too Hard)

The key to sticking with an aerobic exercise programme is to make it fun or interesting. It's often just a matter of finding an activity that you like. Better still, try a mix of activities. Maybe on Mondays you play tennis, Wednesdays you attend an aerobics class, and Fridays you go cycling with your family. But for some women, sticking with one form of exercise is best because they like to excel at one thing. So, for example, if you enjoy running, you may be motivated by constantly trying to improve the time or distance of your runs. As you shop for an aerobic activity that suits your purposes, you'll also learn how to maximise the body-shaping benefits by maximising your effort or frequency.

Another time-honoured aid is to exercise with a friend or family member. If you know someone is going to be there at six in the morning to go for a walk with you, you won't decide you're too tired today and sleep in.

Go cycling with your kids and use the time not only to burn calories but also to talk with them. Or take your husband or partner along on your evening walks, and make the most of this time to yourselves.

Getting Started

Before you start an aerobic exercise programme, ask your doctor for advice if you answer yes to two or more of the following.

- You are over the age of 45.
- You are less than 55 and past menopause and not taking oestrogen-replacement therapy (which protects your heart).
- You smoke cigarettes.
- You have or have ever had high blood pressure or high cholesterol.
- You're sedentary – that is, you work at a desk, have no physically active hobbies or pastimes, or don't currently take regular exercise.
- You have a family history of heart disease, high blood pressure, or high cholesterol.

If your foray into fitness takes you to a health club or other group setting, don't be intimidated by how other women look or whether they are more proficient on treadmills, stairclimbers or various other exercise machines.

Exercise itself will boost your self-esteem. Remember you are there to improve *your* health and well-being. You want to feel good now, and 25 years from now. So this is a commitment to yourself.

Start by gently warming up: walk at an easy pace for 5 minutes to get your blood circulating. Then do some gentle stretches (no bouncing) before you start your aerobic activity. When you've ended your activity, allow your body to cool down. Walk for about 3–5 minutes. Then do some gentle stretches, which will help increase or maintain flexibility.

When starting out, don't be discouraged if you can only do, say, 10 minutes on a particular exercise machine. The next time, lighten the tension and ease the pace and try for 15 minutes. Then try to build upon that gradually.

How much should you increase your performance before levelling off? The rule of thumb is 10 per cent per week, say experts. You can increase either your pace or your time, but you shouldn't increase both at the same time.

For example, say you're walking at 3 miles (4.8km) per hour on a treadmill for 20 minutes at a time, and only sweating lightly. Here are your options: you can increase your time on the machine to 22–23 minutes. Or you can stay at 20 minutes, but increase your speed to 3½–4 miles (5.6–6.4km) per hour. Or you can do neither, but make the degree of incline a little steeper. Do only one increase a week. If you are really enjoying working out, you could keep the intensity and duration the same, but add an extra day. And always take one day off a week, no matter how fit you are.

AEROBICS CLASSES AND VIDEO

Aerobics Stats

Calories Burned*	Body-Shaping Potential
228 per half-hour	Tones abdominals, hips, thighs, buttocks and, depending on type of aerobics performed, also other major muscles

*Based on a 10½ stone (67kg) woman. If you weigh more, you'll burn more calories; if you weigh less, you'll burn fewer.

The fat-blasting, muscle-toning, heart-strengthening moves of aerobics workouts have come a long way since their disco-inspired beginnings. Today's aerobics classes and videos challenge you to kickbox, skip, do tennis swings and more, with background tunes ranging from reggae to golden oldies.

For weight loss, an aerobics workout can hardly be beaten. For muscle toning, aerobics also incorporates resistance exercises that add up to a sleek physique.

Body-Shaping Benefits

Doing aerobics on a regular basis contributes to weight loss and body-toning in several ways:

- You'll burn fat more efficiently.

- You'll tone all your muscles, improving your appearance, strength and stamina.

- You'll improve your flexibility, which extends your range of motion and improves muscle performance, balance and coordination.

Psychological Benefits

Research shows that aerobic exercise imparts increased feelings of well-being and self-confidence while relieving stress, depression, symptoms of PMS and sleep problems.

The Right Gear

Shoes. Shop for trainers, which provide good cushioning, support, flexibility and traction. If you have high-arched feet, look for a shoe with added shock absorption and more ankle support. If your feet tend to be more flat, look for less cushioning and greater support and heel control. For a proper fit, allow ½in (2.5cm) between the end of your longest toe and the end of the shoe. Your shoes should also be as wide as possible across the instep without allowing your heel to slip. A well-fitted shoe does require a breaking-in period. If your feet are blistering after a few days, take the shoes back. Finally, replace your shoes regularly. They lose their cushioning after three to six months of regular use, making you more susceptible to knee and ankle injuries.

Clothes. Look for 'breathable' fabrics in a blend of cotton and synthetic fibres that whisk sweat away from your body, allowing you to keep cool.

If the temperature in your workout area varies, wear a couple of layers that you can take off or put back on as needed.

Videos. Aerobics videos are a great way to exercise at home – you get to enjoy lively music as you follow the moves of other in-shape exercisers bounding across your TV screen. Tapes are available in a wide range of aerobics styles, from traditional choreographed floor aerobics to workouts that help tone specific muscle groups. Consider the following when choosing:

- Type. Look for a workout and music that sparks your personal interest.

- Time. Figure out realistically how long your workout will be. If your time is limited, use 30-minute videos and put a couple of them together at those times when you can do a longer workout. If you're a beginner, decrease the time or the intensity of your routine if it feels too difficult.

■ Intensity. Don't risk discouragement by overestimating what you can do. You're probably a beginner if you haven't even taken a walk for at least six months or you're very overweight. If you walk or do some other form of exercise at least two or three times a week, start at an intermediate level.

Getting Started

Here's what you need to get started and keep going with an aerobics exercise programme.

Learn the basics. Many exercises require a degree of motor skill and coordination, which could take time to develop. Start with an introductory class or videotape workout described as low-impact or no-impact, which means less stress to your joints. As you get used to the programme, gradually move into a more advanced workout.

Warm up. Prepare your body and mind for exercise with a 5–10-minute warm-up of the muscles you will use during your workout. For example, walk on the spot to warm up your legs. Follow with 'static' (gentle with no bouncing) stretching of those same muscles. Warming up helps your body burn calories more efficiently by increasing your core body temperature. It also helps your muscles work faster and more forcefully, improves muscle elasticity and muscle control, and prevents the build-up of pain-provoking lactic acid.

Monitor your intensity level. The talk test is a good, commonsense way to judge whether you're working out at a safe pace. You should be able to carry on a conversation at the same time as exercising. If you can't, slow down.

An aerobics workout will burn fat, strengthen your muscles and help your heart grow stronger as long as you're exercising at a higher than usual heart rate – your 'target heart rate' (see page 166), say experts. If you're just starting out, you want your heart rate during the aerobics portion of your workout to be at the lower end of your target heart rate range. Monitor your pulse rate during your exercise

routine to ensure you don't exceed your maximum heart rate.

Aim for 30–60 minutes. Make it your goal to exercise for at least 30 minutes – either at a single stretch or accumulated throughout the day. If you're an absolute beginner, start out doing only 10–15 minutes during the aerobics portion at a low- to moderate-intensity level. As you grow stronger, gradually add workout time without increasing intensity.

Add toning exercises. Most aerobics classes are followed by a few minutes of exercises specific to muscle strengthening. Look for a class that focuses on your 'problem areas', or add toning exercises with light weights to your home workout.

Cool down. As few as 3 minutes of moderate movement like walking after a workout enables your heart and muscles to return slowly to their normal state. Gentle movements and stretches may also help increase or maintain your flexibility and minimise muscle soreness.

Work out several days a week. In order to lose weight, experts recommend that you exercise at least four or five days a week.

Aerobics Workouts

BEGINNER

10–20 minutes, 3 days a week; target heart rate 60–65 per cent of maximum.

INTERMEDIATE

20–30 minutes, 3–5 days a week; target heart rate 65–75 per cent of maximum.

EXPERIENCED

Minimum 20–30 minutes, 3–5 days a week; target heart rate 75–90 per cent of maximum.

Cycling

If your knees, ankles or hips bother you when you walk, cycling can be a great pain-free way to exercise and lose weight. Unlike walking or running, it isn't a weight-bearing exercise – the bicycle, not your bones and joints, supports your weight.'

Body-Shaping Benefits

Cycling works on you primarily from the hips down. It exercises the muscles in your buttocks, front and back thighs, and lower legs. These are the largest muscles in your body, and when you use them to perform high-intensity work, such as cycling, you burn a lot of calories. So if you bicycle regularly:

- You'll strengthen and tone the muscles of your lower body during your workout.

- You'll burn off a fair amount of stored calories – or fat.

Psychological Benefits

You may well have wonderful memories of exploring your local area by bike as a child, riding with your friends for hours. Yet somewhere along the way – probably once you got your driving licence – your bike started to gather dust in the garage. And that's a shame.

Cycling gets you outside just like walking does, but you can go further. And if you start cycling to work, think of the money you'll save in petrol or fares.

If you typically walk an hour a day for exercise and cover 3–4 miles (4.8–6.4km), you can cycle for the same amount of time and cover 10 miles (16km).

The Right Gear

Shoes and socks. Comfortable, lightweight trainers are fine, as long as the soles have enough grip to stay put on the pedals.

Tuck the laces under the tongue of your shoe so they don't get tangled in the pedals, chain or chain guard. Also, don't tie your laces too tightly, or your feet will fall asleep while you ride. To keep your feet comfortable, choose cotton or cotton-rich socks.

Clothes. Avoid loose-fitting garments, especially on your lower half, as they may chafe with the movement of cycling or, worse, get caught in your chain or handlebars and cause an accident. If you are cycling in traffic you may want to wear a mask to reduce the exhaust fumes you breathe in.

Bike. Even if you have an old one you want to resurrect, you need to take it to a bike shop for a service. It's almost sure to need new tyres and some oil to lubricate the chains and gears.

If you need to buy a bike, you can choose from three types.

- *Road bike.* This kind has drop handlebars (they curve under) and smooth, narrow tyres. They are designed for speed, not comfort.

- *Mountain bike.* These have flat handlebars (they don't curve) and fatter tyres than road bikes. It's easier to balance on them. The tyres are knobby to give better traction. They're designed for riding on rough tracks, over rocks and roots and such – but they function well on tarmac surfaces, too.

■ *Hybrid bike*. These have gears, handlebars and frames similar to mountain bikes, but with narrower tyres to give the smooth ride of a road bike. Bike shops tend to recommend hybrid bikes for adult women.

Fit and comfort are vital. Experts at bike shops are better equipped to measure you and your new equipment than staff at a department store.

■ *The right fit*. Ask for a bike designed especially for women. These have a steeper seat tube (the vertical tube) to position you correctly, and a shorter top tube (running from the seat tube to the head tube and handlebars) to accommodate women's shorter torsos and arms. Or they may steer you towards a man's bike that can be reconfigured to fit you (moving handlebars or changing the seat, for instance, so you don't have to reach as far for the handlebars).

A good fit is essential or your bike will be too uncomfortable to ride regularly. Also, if you're not used to riding a bike with multiple gears you may want to consider one with gears that are clearly numbered, to help you learn how to change them.

■ *A comfortable seat*. Whichever style of bike you choose, you need to feel comfortable in the saddle. You don't want to put pressure on parts of your body that don't respond well to intense friction and excess weight. So do ask about special seats for women. Some feature a wider back and narrower, cut-out nose that takes the weight off delicate tissues for a more comfortable ride. Others use a soft material on the underside with less bracing (used for stiffness) than seats for men's bikes, so that the saddle flexes to absorb impact.

A helmet. Always wear a helmet to protect your head from impact if you collide with the pavement (or anything else). Some helmets are specially designed for women – a big help if, for example, you want to pull your hair back in a ponytail when you ride. Consider a helmet with a vent to help keep you cool, and those with reflective stripes and removable visors for riding at night and in the sun. Wear a cap under your helmet only if the helmet is designed to accommodate one, or you will compromise fit and safety.

Getting Started

Get to know your bike. Before taking off on a long trek, ride around your local area to get to know the gears and brakes on your new equipment.

Practise changing gears. Beginners often stay in one gear. Here's how not to. Technically, the best way to work out whether you're using the right gear for a specific terrain is to count your pedal strokes. To do this, count your pedal revolutions (on one leg) for 15 seconds, then multiply that number by four. Efficient riders do 80–100 revolutions per minute on flat roads, and about 60–85 on hills. Beginners may prefer this easier rule of thumb: use the lower (smaller) gears on steeper terrain and the higher (larger) gears on flatter terrain. Then practise until you get a feel for the combination that enables you to pedal the most efficiently. If you're struggling, change down. If the wheels are spinning with little or no resistance, change up.

Experiment with hand positions. Some hand positions feel better than others. You might feel comfortable riding with your hands close together, while someone else may prefer grasping the very edges of the handlebars.

Follow through when you pedal. Good pedalling involves technique. You have to use your leg muscles on the back end of the pedalling stroke – that is, when you're bringing the pedal back up and bending your leg to pedal efficiently. To do this, imagine you're scraping mud from the bottom of your shoe. In other words, press your leg down, apply force when your foot is at the bottom of the stroke, then use your leg muscles to pull the bottom of your leg back up towards your butt.

Lean forward – or stand – on the hills. As you begin to feel more comfortable, you'll spend more time out of the saddle. For instance, when you go into a turn you'll lean forward out of the seat. When you go up hills you'll stand in order to get more power to your legs.

Watch out for cars, both moving and parked. If you ride on the streets you know you have to look out for moving vehicles. But many street accidents take place when someone who has just parked her car opens the door straight into the path of a bike rider. So keep your eyes and ears open. That means no Walkman.

Take a lesson. Many bike shops offer clinics and classes for novice riders. You'll learn, for example, that, as with driving a car, it's usually best to brake before a turn rather than during one.

Bicycling Workouts

BEGINNER

Cycle non-stop for 20 minutes on flat terrain, 2 or 3 times a week for 3–4 weeks.

INTERMEDIATE

Beginning on flat terrain, cycle fast for 20–30 minutes, then include a couple of hills or change to a harder gear for 5 minutes at a time, without necessarily going fast. Do this 3 times a week until you work your way up to riding comfortably 60 minutes each time.

EXPERIENCED

Extend one of your regularly scheduled rides, probably at the weekend, to at least 1½ times or double the time or distance of a weekday ride. Vary the speed and intensity as you ride: climb hills, ride quickly for a few minutes, and use more intensity at other times.

CYCLING ON AN EXERCISE BIKE

> ## Stationary Cycling Stats
>
> **Calories Burned*** | **Body-Shaping Potential**
>
> 130–330 per half-hour | Tones your leg and butt muscles
>
> ---
>
> **Based on a 10½ stone (67kg) woman. If you weigh more, you'll burn more calories; if you weigh less, you'll burn fewer.*

Many homes have an exercise bike – unused. The trouble is, indoor exercise can be boring. You need to watch TV or listen to music at the same time, or use your bike as an adjunct to another activity. So don't rely on an exercise bike as your sole means of slimming down and shaping up. Think of it as a once- or twice-a-week 'easy workout' to complement regular walking or aerobics.

Body-Shaping Benefits

Here's what you can expect when you use an exercise cycle regularly:

- You'll burn about 5 calories every minute while you exercise. That's a lot more than the single calorie per minute that you burn when you're doing other daily activities.
- You'll develop and strengthen the gluteal muscles in your buttocks, the quadriceps at the front of your thighs and the hamstrings in the back of your thighs.
- There's no impact from your upper-body weight, so you can tone your butt and thigh muscles without putting any stress on your leg joints.

Psychological Benefits

One of the pleasures of stationary cycling is that it's absolutely safe – no wild drivers winging past as you pedal in the quiet of your home, and no risk of hitting a stone and flying head over heels into the gravelly road. So what do with your consciousness while you're pedalling is entirely up to you.

Among your options: put the bike in front of the TV and lose yourself in a video or your

---

Bring Power to Your Pedal

- **Count your miles.** While novice riders simply let their bikes tell them how many revolutions per minute (rpm) they are doing, you can also track the total number of miles you ride. To chart your progress, time yourself over a 'distance' of 10 miles (16km). Keeping the resistance at the same level, ride those 10 miles (16km) again the next time you work out – and see if you can beat your previous time.

- **Design your own programme.** If your bike has an electronic-display programme, you can use that. Or you might design your own programme instead, focusing on resistance (or intensity), heart rate, speed, duration or cadence (the rhythm at which you pedal).

- **Two types of workout.** Sprint work – going fast at a low intensity – helps you work on what are called fast-twitch muscle fibres. Strength work – going slowly at a high intensity – builds the slow-twitch fibres. If you mix and match, you will use a greater number of muscle fibres in different ways, which is more effective than doing the same exercises over and over again.

favourite movie. Catch up with the news or lose yourself in a soap opera while your feet spin. Or place a book or magazine on the front of the cycle if you prefer to read.

The Right Gear

Clothes. The shorts worn by cyclists have extra padding strategically sewn into the crotch and inner-thigh region to make indoor as well as outdoor riding more comfortable.

Bike. A good, new home bike won't be cheap. If money is a problem run an ad for used bikes in your local paper. Whatever you do, sit on the bike and pedal for a while to see how comfortable it is for you. Wear your exercise clothes and trainers. If it doesn't feel right, say no to that bike.

Whether you're buying new or used, here's what to consider.

■ *Upright or recumbent.* Traditional upright bikes aren't designed for women and overweight people in general, because the seats aren't wide enough. And an upright can spell torture if you have lower-back pain. Before you buy, try out a recumbent bike, which has a bucket-shaped seat that supports your back. Or you might like something in-between, called a semi-recumbent.

■ *The right fit.* You should be able to sit up straight on the bike even when pedalling full speed. If you need to hunch over to reach the handlebars, the bike isn't the right size for you.

■ *Adjustability.* No bike is made-to-order, so you need to be able to make adjustments. When you're trying it out, make sure you can move the seat up or down to the right position. When you're seated on an upright bike, your hips should be square on the saddle. At the bottom of the downstroke, with your foot rested firmly on the lower pedal, the extended leg should be slightly bent at the knee. Also, look straight down and see whether you can see your toes. If you can't, you are too far forward, which puts enormous stress on the kneecap. After you

have made all the necessary seat adjustments, check whether the handlebars are still at a comfortable level. If not, adjust them too.

The same criteria apply to a recumbent bike. You should be able to move the seat forward or back, up or down. When it is in the correct position, your extended leg should be slightly bent at the knee.

■ *A gel seat.* Though you may think your hips and butt are well padded, an ordinary bicycle seat can feel like a torture device after many miles of spinning. If you're buying new, ask if you can have a softer gel seat instead of the standard-issue one. If you're getting a used bike, you can find a replacement gel seat at most bicycle or exercise equipment stores.

■ *Upper-body exercise handles.* Rather than normal stationary handlebars, some bikes have handles that you can push and pull, so you'll get some upper-body exercise while your lower limbs are also going full steam ahead. You might enjoy the extra upper-body flex, but movable handles don't increase calorie burning very much and cost extra.

■ *Resistance.* You want to be able to adjust the resistance so that you can vary the intensity of your workouts. On some bikes, resistance is created by a brake pad applying steady pressure. Others use electromagnetic resistance or a fly-wheel. The type of resistance might affect the feel of the bike, but otherwise there is no particular advantage to any of them.

■ *Electronics.* Some bikes have elaborate programmes, along with heart-rate monitors and other devices, to help you measure many different variables. With some, you can race against a computerised competitor. If you like these features and they keep you more challenged, go for them. But they don't affect the operation of the bike or the slimming and trimming benefits you get from it.

■ *Repairs.* Find out how, and where, you can get the bike fixed if something goes wrong. When equipment breaks, workouts come to a standstill.

Getting Started

On an exercise bike, there are, as already mentioned, a number of variables – speed, time, intensity and resistance. Here's how to get them to balance out and keep the challenges reasonable rather than reckless.

Think tempo. Your workout pedalling speed will be affected by the resistance. When the bike is set to the right resistance you should be able to keep a cadence, or rhythm, that is smooth and measured. If the resistance is too great, you'll find yourself pumping your legs to gather momentum for the next turn. If it's set too lightly you'll find yourself pushing and pulling the handlebars, probably with an uneven cadence. The way you pedal should mimic the way you walk when you're striding along at a good pace – a measured and consistent tempo.

Stretch the time, not the heart. When you're starting out, you need to let your legs and heart get used to the pace. At this stage it's better to work out for a longer period at low intensity for a few weeks rather than a short period at high intensity. This will give your heart time to get used to your workouts.

Try some bursts. When you're able to cycle for 20–30 minutes at low to moderate intensity, you can try some short bursts at higher intensity. But don't lose the cadence when you do that. You need to make increases that don't force you to pump too hard or spin too fast.

Vary the resistance. When your feet are spinning and your heart is pumping, it is actually your legs that may first cry for help. In general, most people's leg muscles are weaker than their hearts. If your legs start to feel heavy or sore but you aren't breathing hard, decrease the resistance.

Stationary Cycling Workouts

BEGINNER

Progressive intervals. Over a 22-minute period, intersperse slow-paced, low-intensity riding with short, higher-intensity spurts. Ride at a slow pace and low intensity for 5 minutes, then pedal for 30 seconds at higher intensity. Keep alternating, but end with some slow pedalling to cool down.

Intermediate

Pyramid workout. Ride for 10 minutes at high intensity, then 2 minutes at low intensity. Then do 8 minutes at a level that's even higher than the first 10 minutes – followed by another 2-minute, low-intensity interlude. Each increasingly harder interval should be 2 minutes shorter than the one before, but keep on increasing the intensity – and always insert a 2-minute interval to cool down. The whole routine should take about 40 minutes. Then give yourself some slow pedalling at the end to finish off.

Experienced

Hill training. If you want to test your maximum capacity, ride for a certain amount of time – say, 40 minutes – and use progressively higher resistance throughout. Increase the resistance every 3–4 minutes to increase the intensity of your workout. Halfway through, decrease the resistance at regular intervals over the same amount of time.

DANCING

Dancing Stats

Calories Burned*	Body-Shaping Potential
Per half-hour: ballroom, 105; aerobic, 201–276; modern, 147; line, 150	Tones the muscles of the calves, thighs, abdomen, buttocks, shoulders, arms and upper back

*Based on a 10½ stone (67kg) woman. If you weigh more, you'll burn more calories; if you weigh less, you'll burn fewer.

Dance has ancient roots as a form of celebration, entertainment and courtship and, although it can be vigorous exercise, only recently has it begun to be appreciated for its fitness benefits. People see it as just having fun, but social dance can be as good a workout as playing basketball or running,' says Phil Martin, a dance instructor and lecturer in the department of kinesiology and physical education at California State University in Long Beach. Martin did a study with Dr Betty Rose Griffith to observe the aerobic-conditioning effects of dancing. They found that dancers' heart rates were within their 'exercise benefit zone' (60–85 per cent of estimated maximum heart rate) after doing the samba, the polka, swing dances or the Viennese waltz.

Many folk dances are also highly aerobic. 'You can reach 85 per cent or higher of your maximum heart rate,' Martin notes.

Body-Shaping Benefits

If you dance regularly, you can expect to see these results:

- Your entire lower body will be toned.
- You will strengthen the major muscles of your lower body, including your hamstrings, quadriceps and gluteals. Some dance moves,

such as pulling your partner forward in swing dancing, work the triceps, biceps, deltoids and pectoral muscles.

- You'll lose weight and improve your cardiovascular fitness. Line, folk, jazz, swing, samba, salsa, polka and tap dancing may provide an aerobic workout. Other forms of dance, such as modern dancing or ballet, may be aerobic or not, depending on the moves and tempo.

Psychological Benefits

Dancers tend to be happier and more secure, confident, creative, coordinated, exhilarated, intelligent and energetic than other people. Perhaps this is because dancing requires concentration, creativity and, in most cases, social interaction, which provide health benefits that go beyond the physical ones.

Dance enhances mood, relieves stress and lends variety to life. It can be a way for newcomers or singles to meet people, and a way for married couples to get off their couches and reinvigorate their relationships.

The Right Gear

Since dance is so varied, it's a good idea to call before the first class to be sure your footwear is permitted on the dance floor and your other clothes are appropriate. What you wear on your feet depends on the type of dance you do, though modern dance is often done barefoot. When purchasing dance shoes (excluding tennis shoes), go to a specialist shop where you can be fitted by an expert. Here are some things to look for when you choose.

Tennis shoes. For social dancing, you'll need a pair of shoes that turn easily on the floor without being too slippery. Generally, a tennis shoe with some padding is a good idea if you plan to dance all evening, since your feet may burn the next day from the constant impact. If you find that the studio or stage where you dance is sticky, you may need a leather- or suede-soled shoe.

Ballroom shoes. These are ideal because they have suede soles that allow you to glide and turn but aren't too slippery. The rest of the shoe is usually made out of leather, which is lightweight and flexible. However, they are expensive. Keep the shoes clean with a shoe polish brush. Wax build-up on the soles can cause them to harden and lose friction.

Cowboy boots. For line dancing you can wear tennis shoes or, for greater authenticity, cowboy boots. Low heels and natural materials will keep you cool and comfortable.

Ballet shoes. These should be somewhat snugger than street shoes because they are soft and will stretch. Your toe should touch the end when you're standing flat, but it should not be scrunched. If the shoes are too roomy, the leather will crinkle when you stand on your toes. Make sure you buy shoes that accommodate both the width and the length of your foot.

Tap shoes. Jazz tap shoes are available in various styles. Go for low-heeled as a beginner, since it is harder to learn in a high-heeled shoe.

Socks. These should keep your shoes on without your feet slipping, but shouldn't make your shoes too snug, since your feet may swell during an evening on the dance floor. Socks that have cotton or cotton blends help reduce slipping because they reduce sweat.

Clothing. Modern and ballet dancers generally wear comfortable leotards, tights and perhaps leg warmers. Square dancers and folk dancers may wear costumes, while line dancers wear jeans and Western shirts. Aerobic and jazzercise dancers wear fitness clothing, such as exercise bras, leggings and shorts.

Social dancing is generally done in casual street clothing, not exercise wear. Women shouldn't wear slippery fabric that may slide out of their partners' grasp or belts that could catch on an outstretched hand.

Getting Started

Because you can easily reach your maximum heart rate when you dance, it's a good idea to consult your doctor before you start. To find beginners' dance classes in your area, look in your local newspaper, telephone book, public library or town hall.

Start simple. Some dances are easy to learn. You may want to begin with a class that features cha cha, salsa or mambo, and rumba. If you're a real couch potato, you could start with a nice, slow fox-trot.

Take it slow. Until you learn the steps, you may not feel you're getting a workout. Don't worry – your concentration now will pay off in major fitness benefits within a few weeks.

Spice your workout with variety. Remember: one dance will not tone every muscle, increase your strength and flexibility, and provide a fat-burning aerobic workout. So mix and match. Remember that the speed of the music and your own energy level makes a lot of difference.

Play, stop, rewind. If you love the idea of dancing but are too shy to learn with others, brush up on the important steps at home by watching dance videos. Then you can join a class with confidence.

Dancing Workouts

BEGINNER

Try a class that offers a slow waltz, foxtrot or rumba. Dance at a level that allows easy conversation.

INTERMEDIATE

Dance the Viennese waltz, samba or salsa.

EXPERIENCED

Do the polka, jitterbug or line dance.

ELLIPTICAL TRAINING

Elliptical Training Stats

Calories Burned*	Body-Shaping Potential
500–600 per hour	Tones muscles of the entire lower body and burns fat

*Based on a 10½ stone (67kg) woman. If you weigh more, you'll burn more calories; if you weigh less, you'll burn fewer.

An elliptical trainer is about as close as anything comes to a perfect exercise machine. It looks like a combination of treadmill, cross-country ski machine and stepping machine, and it combines the movements (and benefits) of hiking, cross-country skiing and cycling. Your feet move, not back and forth, but in an oval (or elliptical) pattern.

The elliptical trainer is versatile: you can use it to climb or glide. You get a calorie-burning workout that pumps your heart like an all-out run but without stress and strain on your joints – the ideal routine for overweight women who can't jog. Even though most women burn hundreds of calories on it, they feel as if they're just strolling. So you can get rid of unwanted accumulations of fat on your belly, butt or thighs without having to push yourself as hard as on other machines.

Body-Shaping Benefits

Here's what you can expect when you use an elliptical trainer regularly.

- When you move forward you'll work your quadriceps (the big muscles on the front of your thighs) and gluteus muscles (that shape your backside).
- You'll tone and slim your entire lower body.
- You'll notice that your legs are shapelier than

ever, since elliptical training uses all the muscles of the legs, large and small.

- You'll burn approximately 10 calories per minute while you work, and you'll continue to burn calories at a higher rate for a few hours afterwards.

Psychological Benefits

If you have tried treadmill running and found it boring, or if you're ready for a change, the easy-to-use elliptical trainer offers varied programmes to keep you moving for a long time to come.

The Right Gear

Shoes and socks. Because your feet don't leave the machine's surface, any lightweight athletic shoe will do. But don't tie the laces too tightly or your feet will start to feel numb. To keep your feet dry and blister-free, pair those shoes up with athletic-wear socks in cotton or another breathable material.

Clothes. As with most workouts, your best bet is a layer or two of loose-fitting, comfortable clothing in fabrics that wick sweat away. That way, you can peel off a layer as you work up a sweat.

The right machine. An elliptical trainer has various settings: resistance, speed and, usually, ramp. You can programme just one setting at a time, or all three together.

As with an ordinary exercise bike, resistance on an elliptical trainer determines how much effort it will take for you to keep your feet moving. Ramp levels describe how high or low you've set the angle of the ellipse. For instance, a high ramp mimics hiking, while a low ramp mimics cross-country skiing. As you move, you determine the speed at which you move on the trainer. The resistance will, of course, affect the speed at which you *can* move, but how you respond to the resistance is under your control. You could, for example, choose a low resistance and move quickly, or you could put the resistance up high and not be able to move smoothly. Ideally you should move at a comfortable, moderate speed, interspersed with occasional bursts of high intensity as well as high speeds.

Quality elliptical trainers may cost up to six times as much as a treadmill or exercise bike, putting them out of range for many people. So you'll probably use a trainer at a gym or fitness centre, at least to start with. If you fall in love with elliptical training and do want to buy a home machine, here are some buying tips from experts.

■ *Go for range.* Look for a variety of ramp settings and intensity levels. If the ellipse itself isn't expansive and doesn't offer ramp and intensity changes, the workout isn't nearly as effective. If you can afford it, consider a model with a control panel that offers various pre-programmed courses and records how many calories you've burned.

■ *Skip the handles.* Some machines come with handles that allow you to move your arms back and forth – with resistance – while you're on the elliptical machine, but that doesn't increase calorie burning very much. It's more effective to buy a machine without handles and work your legs at a higher intensity without leaning on your arms.

■ *Try various settings.* As with a treadmill or exercise bike, you'll want to know how the machine feels at different settings. So try different combinations of ramp and speed settings and vary the resistance, which enables you to work at different levels of intensity. The higher the resistance, the more power you'll need to exert to get your feet moving.

■ *Measure twice, buy once.* Elliptical trainers are big – up to 5ft (1.5m) long and over 4ft (1.2m) tall. Before you buy, measure the space in which you plan to use the machine.

Getting Started

People with lower-back problems may find this kind of exercise jarring, so consult your doctor before working out on an elliptical trainer. When you first step on to an elliptical trainer, you'll probably start going backwards, which tends to be the natural movement. That's fine for a minute or two, but going backwards doesn't work the legs as effectively as forward motion. You will burn slightly more calories by going in reverse, but not enough to justify the strain on your knees.

A Workout with Options Galore

• **Cross-country skiing motion.** To simulate cross-country skiing (basically, just walking on skis), set the ramp level on low. This exercise uses the butt and hamstring muscles. Try to keep the pace and resistance level moderate, so that you can move smoothly.

• **Hiking motion.** If you want to stay in shape for weekend hiking, or if you just want the benefits that hiking brings to your quadriceps and butt, keep the ramp setting on high and increase the intensity, which will simulate climbing.

• **Jogging motion.** If you keep the ramp setting at middle height you'll get a motion that is close to running, but you won't suffer the same impact on your knees.

• **Put it all together.** With so many options, you can mix and match ramp and intensity levels to create all types of workouts. For instance, you could move from sport to sport within one workout, or do a different sport each time you get on the equipment. Either way, your lower body reaps an amazing array of benefits.

Instead, simply place your feet on the foot pads and push forward slightly. The trainer will begin to move your legs in the elliptical shape; all you have to do is follow. The higher the level of resistance, the harder you'll have to push.

Go slowly. While you may be tempted to power your way through the virtual hills and valleys over which the elliptical machine can take you, stay in the mid-range at first. Once you are used to the machine you can increase something every week, but not two things at once. For example, in the second week you could increase the number of times you exercise from two to three. In the third week you might increase your intensity. In the fourth you could increase from 10 to 20 minutes. And make sure you include other kinds of aerobic activity in your weekly exercise routine.

Keep your hands free. Getting your balance can be tricky at first. But you'll burn far more calories if you let go of the handles, so let your arms swing freely or try a little pumping action.

Keep your head straight. You may get distracted and look around or talk to someone, but twisting your torso is a no-no. To keep your knees in line with your feet and avoid injury, always point your head straight forward.

Elliptical Training Workouts

BEGINNER

2 or 3 times a week for 10–20 minutes at a time in a slow rhythm.

INTERMEDIATE

2 or 3 times a week for at least 20 minutes, using a pre-programmed workout that doesn't include intervals.

EXPERIENCED

2 or 3 times a week, for 20–60 minutes of interval training, either pre-programmed or self-directed.

GARDENING

Stretching, repetition and even resistance principles similar to those of weight training, are involved in gardening, and you also expend calories. Besides making it easier to lose weight and keep it off, helping your garden grow can reduce your risk of heart disease, diabetes, colon cancer and high blood pressure as well as build stronger and healthier bones, muscles and joints.

Body-Shaping Benefits

Gardening provides excellent whole-body exercise. Here's how.

- Walking and other large-muscle movements provide an aerobic workout. Gardening activities like raking, sweeping, hoeing and shovelling are the most aerobic because they are sustained activities.

- You'll exercise your back, chest, abdomen, buttocks, legs, arms and shoulders with the pushing and pulling movements of digging and raking. Your arms and shoulders will get exercise as you plant and weed, and prune bushes and trees. Finally, you'll exercise your legs and buttocks with the repetitive up-and-down of moving along a flower or vegetable bed as you work.

- Gardening offers the kind of sustained, moderate, fat-burning workout that, when performed three to five times a week, can help you lose weight and stay that way.

The Right Gear

Shoes. Because of the many positions your feet will adopt as you garden, you'll need shoes with flexible toes and rear-foot support. Consider gardening clogs, which can be very comfortable for certain foot types. For heavy work, walking shoes or biking boots are safest.

Clothes. What you wear can make all the difference. In warmer weather wear loose-fitting lightweight clothes that will breathe when you perspire. In cooler weather, dress in layers that you can easily take off and put back on as necessary. Don't forget thick gloves to keep soil and prickles at bay.

Tools. Manual tools that you have to push or pull will build strong legs while you firm your abdomen and buttocks. A push lawnmower instead of a ride-on, or an old-fashioned rake instead of a motorised leaf-blower, will help give you the workout you're looking for. When buying tools like clippers or edgers, choose manual not electric versions. Pay particular attention to ergonomics: look for comfortable handles and angles that require effort yet don't put undue strain on your back or other parts of your body.

Other stuff. Find yourself a cushiony mat you can kneel or sit on while weeding. Don't forget to wear sunscreen and a hat to ward off damaging ultraviolet rays (yes, even in Britain!).

Getting Started

If you have a large plot of land to work with, first warm up by taking a brisk walk around your property. Breathe in the fresh air and take in the wonders of nature all around you. This helps prepare you for the effort and makes you less prone to injuries. For details on how to stretch, see Chapter 10. But size isn't everything. Cultivating your green fingers in a 'container garden' outside your back door is good too.

Either way, here's how to get started.

Set reasonable goals. Don't expect to dig and plant your garden all at once. Do one thing at a time, a little at a time.

Choose the right time. During hot weather, go inside between 10 a.m. and 2 p.m.. Also, try working when you're usually most energetic. If you're a morning person, start when the sun comes up. If you don't get revved up until later in the day, save gardening for the late afternoon or evening.

Drink plenty of water. To avoid dehydration, which can lead to fatigue and muscle cramp, have a glass of water before you begin gardening, and sip frequently from a jug or water bottle while you're out there.

Aim for variety. Engaging in a variety of movements every time you garden trains a variety of muscles, making you stronger and more toned overall. It also reduces the risk of overstressing specific muscles and joints. For example, dig for 10 minutes, then switch to planting or weeding, then to watering, and then to tossing weeds and rubbish into a bag.

Switch sides. Give the muscles on both sides of your body a good workout. For example, rake from the left, then from the right, and keep alternating . Otherwise you'll end up out of balance, with one side of your body noticeably stronger than the other. There's also more risk of muscle strain if you stick to one side.

Bend and lift carefully. Gardening can put a real strain on your lower back. Instead of bending at the waist to weed or plant, squat down on one knee, with the other knee bent. When lifting, use your legs instead of your back.

Hold tools up close. Even the lightest tools

Gardening Keeps Kate Slim and Young

Kate lost 25lb (11.4kg) and looks more like 39 than 49 – thanks to gardening, her favourite form of 'exercise'.

'During my childhood and young adult years I'd always been self-conscious about my weight,' says clinical therapist and single mum Kate. 'All my female relatives were chubby, and I saw myself gaining weight and starting to look just like them.'

Kate tried running, aerobics and even walking, but for differing reasons had no success. Then she bought a little house with a garden for herself and her boys, and plunged into gardening in a big way – with big results.

'I was determined to make the most of the space – I ripped out parts of the lawn and planted beds of medicinal herbs, shrubs and ornamental grasses, plus a few vegetables. There are three of us, but you know how kids feel about vegetables and gardening,' she adds.

In summer, Kate gets up early to garden. 'I start out with easy stuff, like pulling weeds, then do some planting, and stop before it gets hot,' she says. 'I get some exercise every single day during the growing season.'

Make no mistake about it, says Kate: gardening is a real workout. 'I'm moving constantly – yanking weeds, carrying buckets of mulch and clippings, raking the soil flat.'

For Kate exercise, not dieting, is the key to staying in shape. 'I have the metabolism of a snail, so being active is the only answer for me. And when you get some exercise, you feel you "earn" what you eat and don't feel guilty about every single bite.'

can strain your muscles when they're used for the repetitive motions of gardening. To reduce the strain, hold tools closer to your body. Rather than stretching for weeds and placing your back in an unsupported position, dig up the ones that are nearby with a small trowel or fork held close to your side. Then either switch sides after you've pulled out all the weeds that are close to you, or do one side of a row and then come back down the other side. To include more stretching while gardening, reach with your whole torso, making sure your back is supported under your feet and legs.

Stop when you're tired. Don't be a weekend warrior, working in your garden from dawn till dark Saturday and aching from head to toe on Sunday. Instead, spread your gardening out over the entire weekend. Better yet, spread it out over several days throughout the week.

Gardening Workouts

BEGINNER

Weeding or planting seeds or seedlings for 10 minutes at a time.

INTERMEDIATE

Tilling with a long-handled tiller, or hoeing or other chores for 30 minutes at a time.

EXPERIENCED

Digging or spreading fertiliser or mulch or other chores for 45 minutes at a time, 5 days a week

HIKING

Hiking Stats

Calories Burned*	Body-Shaping Potential
250 per half-hour	Tones the legs and buttocks; will also increase aerobic endurance

*Based on a 10½ stone (67kg) woman. If you weigh more, you'll burn more calories; if you weigh less, you'll burn fewer.

Breathe deeply. Enjoy the view, smell the clean air, listen to the skylarks.

Hiking is like walking but with one major difference: it takes you to new and exciting landscapes. So if you have been walking or running and hanker for variety, take to the hills and long-distance footpaths.

Body-Shaping Benefits

Physiologically, hiking is walking turned up a notch or two. Here's how you can benefit.

- You'll burn more calories by hiking than by walking, since climbing hills or walking on uneven ground takes more energy.

- When you carry a pack of some kind (which most people do), the extra weight further pumps up your calorie burning.

- You'll give your quadriceps, hamstrings, gluteus maximus and gluteus minimus (the major muscles in your hips, thighs, and buttocks) a good workout, since hill walking forces your leg and thigh muscles to work harder and more intensely than walking on the flat.

- If you use hiking poles, you'll tone your arm and back muscles, too.

The Right Gear

Footwear. For short hikes on relatively flat ground you can get by with running or walking shoes. But in general your feet will be a lot happier in hiking boots, especially if you have problems with weak ankles or balance. Look for boots with lugged rubber soles to provide traction over rocks, soil, leaves and tree roots, all of which are slippery, especially when wet. Make sure they are big enough to accommodate thick socks (see below).

Socks. If you're going on a long hike – more than half a day or so – wear two pairs of socks. The first (closest to your feet) should be made in lightweight material that wicks away moisture. The outer layer should be of a thicker material that protects your feet from rubbing against your shoe, like wool. For greater comfort change both pairs halfway through your trip.

Clothes. Thinking jeans? Think again. Cotton holds moisture against the skin if it gets wet from inside or outside the body. Instead, go to a specialist sports or climbing gear shop to buy nylon shorts or hiking trousers and pullovers made from fabrics such as polypropylene, which keep moisture away from your body and dry quickly. In extremely cold weather, wear three layers. Use fabrics such as polypropylene as an inner layer to wick moisture away from the skin. As a middle layer, insulate by trapping a layer of warm air next to your body with fleece or wool. The outer layer should shield you from weather extremes: wind jackets and trousers of either Gore-Tex or Gore-Tex and fleece are good outer protectors. If the weather is clear and only mildly cold, an inner and middle layer will be enough. Finally, if it's cool enough to wear a jacket you also need gloves and a hat, since the greatest source of heat loss is through the head and other extremities.

Food. If you're heading out for a couple of hours or longer, count on getting hungry. Take snacks that are high in complex carbohydrates, such as cereal bars, dried fruit, bananas or a sandwich.

Water. Any time you exercise for an hour or more, you need to drink water to avoid even mild dehydration. So always carry bottled water or a water purifier. Never drink water from a stream because you don't know what might be upstream. Waste from livestock or wildlife, or even decomposing animals could be nearby.

Walking stick. You can buy one, or simply use a sturdy stick you find on your hike. Walking sticks are great if you have a back problem, bad knees or trouble with balance. It's like a third leg. Experienced hikers prefer two hiking poles. They also come in handy when crossing small streams, and when you are going downhill help to lessen the impact on the knees.

A map. Unless you can see the entire area that you're walking *while* you're walking, you need a map on the appropriate scale. For longer trips a compass may be called for.

Other potentially useful items. Just in case something goes wrong, consider packing a torch and a small, basic first aid kit. And, especially if you're going off the beaten track, tell someone responsible where you're going and when you intend to be back.

Getting Started

You'll enjoy hiking more – and you'll be less likely to feel sore the next day – if you get yourself in practice.

Practise on stairs. The one type of walk you can't practise for in a gym is going downhill, so make use of any long stairs to get your quadriceps and knees ready for the descents.

Practise with your pack and poles. Your bag or briefcase may weigh a ton, but how often do you sling them behind you and carry them up hills for seven or eight hours? If you're preparing for a long hike, load up your pack

when you're going short distances. You'll find out just how much weight you're comfortable with, and get to know the ins and outs of your pack.

Practise with your poles, too – it takes time to get used to using them before you can build up speed.

Adjust your stride. When you walk on flat ground, you tend to take long strides. But hiking requires small steps if you are to remain steady on uneven ground.

Hiking a mile on a trail isn't the same as walking the same distance on the flat. Distances can be deceptive. So pay attention to guidebook estimates of how long a trail is, the elevation gained and how much time it takes.

Tips for Hikers

Hiking isn't a race. If anything it's leisurely, because even when the terrain is challenging you're taking time to notice just how beautiful nature is.

Hiking Workouts

BEGINNER

20–30 minutes of hiking on a trail or on a beach 3 times a week.

INTERMEDIATE

40 minutes of hiking 5 or 6 days a week, plus a long hike (60 minutes) up and over a steep hill on day 7.

EXPERIENCED

Longer hikes on rockier terrain, which take 2–4 hours; for highly experienced hikers, trips that last longer than 4 hours.

HOUSEWORK

Housework Stats

Calories Burned*	Body-Shaping Potential
30–50 per 10-minute period	Tones arms, shoulders, chest, back, buttocks, abdomen and legs

*Based on a 10½ stone (67kg) woman. If you weigh more, you'll burn more calories; if you weigh less, you'll burn fewer.

They're the words you've been waiting to hear: cleaning your house counts as exercise!

Health and fitness experts agree that the everyday exercise of picking up dirty socks, scrubbing floors and slaving over a hot stove qualifies as just the moderately intense sort of physical activity you need to stay healthy and fit.

'It may seem that spending 15–20 minutes vacuuming a couple of rooms doesn't come to much, but in the long term people who do quite a lot of housework will reap significant benefits in terms of calorie expenditure, fitness and health,' says South Carolina exercise physiologist, Dr Russell Pate.

Body-Shaping Benefits

Because it engages all your major muscle groups housework builds strength, endurance and flexibility. Here's how.

- Picking up clutter and carrying it from one room to another and – an even greater challenge – carrying it up and down stairs works the muscles of your arms, shoulders, legs and buttocks while your back and abdominal muscles stabilise your body.

- You'll primarily work your upper body by pushing a vacuum cleaner, but walking with your cleaner from one end of your home to the other works your legs and mid-section.

- Scrubbing a floor or cleaning windows helps maintain strength in your arms and back,

Say Goodbye to Your Cleaner – And Shape Up

In her late forties Julie became determined to start exercising regularly. She had put on weight during the menopause and felt awfully out of shape.

She first went to a health club to which her daughter had given her a one-year membership. 'I went once, but I hated it,' she recalls. 'You have to dress, get organised, drive to the place, find a parking spot, get undressed, put on your workout clothes, get into step with everybody else in class, then undress again, shower . . . all that!'

At just about the same time, her cleaner retired, so Julie decided to reclaim her mop and vacuum cleaner and set about turning cleaning her house into an exercise regime.

'I have three storeys to vacuum,' she says, 'plus wooden floors everywhere to mop. I'm constantly picking things up and climbing up and down stairs to put them away. I have lots of windows to wash, and when I do I stretch as much as I can and alternate arms. When I'm doing laundry I throw everything on the floor. Then I sort it all out with a kind of ballet movement, bending down for each piece and throwing it in a sweeping motion. There's always housework to be done, so I may as well get the most out of it.' She does occasional cleaning all week long, then a once-a-week major clean.

'It really is a wonderful way to stay in shape,' Julie says. 'I'm 61 and I feel better than I did in my forties.'

while the stretching motion maintains your flexibility.

- You can make almost any everyday chore aerobic by aiming to reach your target heart rate zone. Just monitor your heart rate while you work. Start with about 50 per cent of your estimated maximum heart rate (see page 166 for the formula). As you build endurance, gradually push yourself to higher levels. Work faster, or without stopping and starting. But don't exceed 85–90 per cent of your maximum heart rate.

Getting Started

Anyone who has spent a weekend spring-cleaning only to wake up stiff and sore on Monday morning knows that certain precautions are called for:

Take it slow. Work yourself up gradually to doing housework for extensive periods, especially strenuous tasks.

Start your day with stretches. Honestly, now, are any of us likely to stop and stretch our hamstrings before laying hands on a broom? The most practical alternative is a simple stretching routine every morning when you get out of bed.

Alternate activities. To avoid overworking particular muscles, switch from one task to another. Move the work around to different muscle groups and move the stress around from joint to joint and tissue to tissue. For example, do some vacuuming, then put in a load of laundry, then clean the bathroom.

Perceive your exertion. If you've been sedentary and now want to tackle your housework with fervour, pay attention to how you feel every step of the way. Exercise experts call this 'rating your perceived exertion'. If you start to feel tired or short of breath, slow down and turn to a less strenuous activity.

Position yourself properly. The bending, lifting, twisting, reaching and other often demanding movements of housework can play havoc with muscles and joints. Don't force yourself into positions you're not accustomed to or that feel abnormal. And certainly don't do so over and over again or for a long period of time.

For instance, don't get down on your hands and knees to scrub the floor for 30 minutes if you're not used to being in that position. Instead, ease into it for a few minutes, then switch to another task and come back to the floor later – if you feel OK. And avoid stretching yourself into postures befitting a contortionist to reach beneath the sofa or behind the fridge.

Bend and lift carefully. Housework can put a real strain on your vulnerable lower back. Bend and lift with your legs, not your back.

Think, '30 minutes a day'. Weight-loss experts recommend 30 minutes or more of moderately intense physical activity daily. That's a brisk walk or its equivalent. Pushing a vacuum cleaner, washing windows, scrubbing floors could be the equivalent.

As with any other form of exercise, if you've been sedentary up to now start out with 10–15 minutes of housework two or three days a week and build from there.

Housework Workouts

LOW INTENSITY

Doing laundry, making beds, ironing, washing dishes, putting away groceries, cooking, vacuuming.

MODERATE INTENSITY

Sweeping out the garage, cleaning windows, mopping vigorously.

HIGH INTENSITY

Moving household furniture, carrying heavy boxes, climbing or carrying items upstairs.

JOGGING AND TREADMILL RUNNING

Jogging Stats

Calories Burned*	Body-Shaping Potential
102 per mile	Firms the calves, thighs, buttocks and, to a lesser extent, the abdomen

*Based on a 10½ stone (67kg) woman. If you weigh more, you'll burn more calories; if you weigh less, you'll burn fewer.

Jogging gives you more value for your money than walking, since it uses the same muscle groups but burns calories faster.

You will burn about 100 calories a mile. Walking one mile may take you 15–20 minutes; jogging will take you half as long. Simply defined as running slowed down, jogging offers less risk of injury than full-out running while providing top-notch aerobic benefits.

Body-Shaping Benefits

Whether you jog on a treadmill or in a park, you will get a wealth of physical payoffs.

- You work both the large and the small muscle groups of your calves, thighs, buttocks and hips, and in a less pronounced way your waist and abdominal muscles.

- You burn calories and use up fat stores.

- You'll keep your metabolic rate raised even after your running shoes are back in the cupboard. According to researchers at the University of Colorado, the resting metabolic rates of middle-aged women runners stayed steady as they grew older, while sedentary women gained weight and body fat as their resting metabolisms slowed. In the long run, older runners burn up to 600 additional calories a week (equal to 9lb/4kg a year!) even when they're at rest. And that doesn't include the calories burned when they run.

The Right Gear

Fortunately for joggers, manufacturers now design shoes to accommodate the sizes and running styles of virtually any woman, at a range of prices. Here's what to look for.

Shoes for *your* feet. Go to a specialist sporting goods stores and take your old shoes along. Worn spots show whether you run more on the outside or the inside of your foot and which areas need the most support.

Enough wiggle room. A wide toebox is vital to give the front of your foot enough room when it is pushed forward.

All-weather, all-surface tread and materials. If you're going to be running in rain and snow, look for a shoe made from weatherproof fabric, with a hard-core outer tread. If you're a treadmill runner, this isn't important.

Replacements, as needed. Buy a new pair of shoes every six months or 600 miles (1000km). At that point the shoes start to fall apart, even if they still look good. You can prolong the life of your running shoes by wearing them only to run.

Treadmill Tips

If you find that rain, sleet and snow keep you from jogging, try treadmill running at a gym. If you like it and can afford it, consider a treadmill for your home. To save money, look in the small ads in your local paper.

Choose a body-friendly model. Some treadmills have built-in suspension, like shock absorbers on a car, to minimise the impact on weak hips or knees. These machines approximate the impact of running on a soft surface. They're also sturdier and better able to accommodate heavier walkers and runners than lightweight units that you can stow under a bed.

Make It Fun

If jogging is your sport of choice, but you have trouble getting out there as often as you'd like – or you're starting to get bored – make it more fun. Here are some tips.

• **Vary your route**. If you run outdoors, change your route often, run with friends or make it a family activity.

• **Run for charity.** The next time you see a charity run announced in the newspaper, sign up. The opportunity to raise money for causes like breast cancer, arthritis or Alzheimer's research (and the free T-shirt) will motivate you to stick with your programme.

Go for a test jog. If you decide to buy, go to a reputable fitness showroom dressed for action. Run on many treadmills, looking for a shock-absorbing platform plus a belt wide and long enough for your comfort and handrails you like.

Know you can stop. So you can stop without risking injury, make sure the treadmill has a device that will immediately stop the belt if you run into trouble.

Getting Started

Unless you're already in shape, work up to jogging gradually. Start out walking, then increase their distance and then their intensity.

Jog at a slow pace for 10, then 15, then 20 minutes, making sure you're not so out of breath that you can't talk to a partner while running. When you're ready for more, run longer, not faster.

If you've been jogging faithfully at a leisurely pace – about 6 miles (10km) per hour – and you're not seeing the results you're looking for, your best bet is to increase your distance, not your speed.

You don't need to run every day. Running too fast – or too often – can increase the risk of knee, hip or tendon problems, or other common injuries (see below for recommended times and distances). There are better ways to maximise your efforts. Here's how.

Increase your weekly distance by no more than 10 per cent a week. If you're jogging three days a week for 30 minutes a day, for example, and covering 3 miles (5km), increase by no more than one mile (0.6km) in total the first week.

Stick to flat, smooth surfaces. If you run outdoors, you can run longer while minimising impact if you use a soft, smooth, unbanked cinder track or an artificial surface.

Alternate jogging with other activities. Swimming, water aerobics, cycling, climbing stairs or using a rowing machine give your feet and legs a welcome respite from the constant pounding of running, and work other muscle groups than running does alone.

Jogging Workouts

BEGINNER

Alternate jogging and walking for 20 minutes a day, 3–5 days a week.

INTERMEDIATE

Jog 40 minutes at least 4 or 5 days a week.

EXPERIENCED

Jog for an hour, up to 5 times a week, not to exceed 30 miles (48km) a week. Beyond that distance, there is really no extra benefit, and your risk of injury increases.

POWER WALKING

Power Walking Stats

Calories Burned*	Body-Shaping Potential
Between 198 and 250 per mile	Tones hips, thighs, buttocks and abdominals

*Based on a 10½ stone (67kg) woman. If you weigh more, you'll burn more calories; if you weigh less, you'll burn fewer.

If you're like a lot of women who walk to lose weight and get in shape, you've probably been walking around your local area religiously for months. You know every child, cat and dog. You're out there, rain or shine. There's just one problem: you're getting bored. You don't want to jog, but you would like to burn a few more calories or get slimmer sooner.

Power walking is the sport for you. It is any walking done as exercise, rather than just recreation. While the average walker usually covers about 3 miles (5km) in an hour-long walk, a power walker strives to do at least 4 miles (6.4km). Serious power walkers can do about 6 miles (10km) an hour – faster than some people run.

Body-Shaping Benefits

Here's what you can expect when you power walk regularly.

- You burn calories in less time.
- You will tone all the muscles in your lower body, including the gluteus (the large muscle in your buttocks), hamstrings (along the backs of your thighs) and quadriceps (in the fronts of your thighs).

The Right Gear

Shoes. Look for lightweight walking shoes that breathe (with mesh on the top or sides).

The upper should be flexible, so it bends fairly easily. A slanted or bevelled heel makes it easier to walk with a heel-to-toe motion and puts less strain on your shin muscles, thus avoiding shin splints. Try on lots of pairs until you find the shoes that are most comfortable for you.

Fresh air or treadmill. The difference between an ordinary walker and a power walker is technique. For starters, you'll want to know exactly how long your training ground is. You can map out a course that's 4–5 miles (6.4–8km) long, do laps on a local athletics track or walk on a treadmill that records your pace and distance automatically. Each of these choices has its own benefits.

Walking through a park or your neighbourhood can be wonderful because of the scenery and varying terrain. Tracks are good because you can concentrate on technique and don't have to worry about traffic. Both enable you to breathe fresh air. Treadmills, on the other hand, tell you about your pace and distance, which is very helpful in the beginning (but remember that you aren't getting the benefits of fresh air).

Water. Carry a water bottle with you. Power walks are more intense than ordinary walks, so it's important to have water before, during and after your workout. Drink at least one glass before starting out, a glass or more while you're walking, and still more water afterwards.

Carry a bottle of water in your hand or buy a suitable waist pack.

A progress log. Metamorphosing from a walker to a power walker means keeping track of your progress. Just write down when you walked, how far you went, how it felt and how long it took you.

Heart rate monitor. These devices, available at sporting goods stores, give a much more accurate reading than you would get from taking your own pulse manually.

Getting Started

Focus on your feet, your hips and your arms.

Warm up first. Walk at a comfortable pace for about 5 minutes or until you break out in a light sweat. Then stretch your quadriceps, hips, hamstrings and shins.

To hone your power-walking technique you'll need to focus on your feet, your hips and your arms.

Feet: think heel-toe. Take quick, short steps, not long, extended strides. Your goal is to pick up your feet faster so you have to focus on rolling your foot from heel to toe. Come down on your heel, with your toes up, then roll through your foot, pushing off on your toes when that leg is behind you. It should almost feel as if you're rolling forward.

Hips: think steady and straight. Your hips are used as an extension of your legs, so each hip moves forward and back (but stays level) as its accompanying leg moves forward. You're not pushing your hips but utilising their power.

Arms: think propulsion. Your arms play a big role in how fast you walk. The faster you pump your arms, the faster your body will move. But don't swing your arms wildly. Your arms should be bent at a 90-degree angle and move steadily forward and back, but your fists should never go further back than your hips or higher than your breastbone.

Eyes: look ahead. Aim for a landmark far ahead of you. That focus will add to your momentum as well as making sure that your posture is correct.

Posture: lean forward from the ankles. Imagine yourself looking like a ski jumper in midair. In other words, there should be no bend in your waist.

Do it to music. If you're just beginning to change your walk into a power walk, you might need music with 110 beats per minute, which is a 19-minute-per-mile pace – just a tad faster than the usual 3-mile-an-hour pace!

If you're doing a solid power walk, pick music with 130 beats per minute, which translates to a 15-minute-per-mile pace.

If you're going full throttle at the breakneck speed of 13-minutes-per-mile, pick music with 150 beats per minute.

Whole body: stretch afterwards. Power walking is hard on many lower-body parts, so make sure you stretch properly afterwards.

Concentrate on hips, quadriceps, hamstrings and shins. Shin pain is common among fitness walkers. Ideally, your shins should adjust to a walk within the first 5 minutes. If they hurt or ache, you're going too fast. Slow down or try walking backwards (retro-walking), which takes all the pressure off the shins. Once your shins feel better, walk forwards again.

Speed, not haste. Only attempt to move through the three intensity workouts detailed here if you're already an experienced walker. That means you are already walking at least three, and possibly more, days per week. Each of your walks should include a 5-minute walking warm-up, 25 minutes of moderate-intensity walking and then a 5-minute walking cool-down, plus some stretching. Then focus on technique followed by speed. When that feels right, start increasing the distance you go at that intensity.

When exercising at high intensity, your goal is to work at 80–90 per cent of your maximum heart rate for the longest portion of your workout, while keeping your technique as flawless as possible.

Power Walking Workouts

BEGINNER

Using power-walking techniques, start to change the way you move during your walk. Bend your arms at a 90-degree angle, pump them, and try to walk heel-to-toe. Do this once or twice during your regular walks for a few weeks before moving on to the next level.

Intermediate

Start working intervals into your routine, using landmarks as your goals. Then give yourself plenty of time to recover (using a slower walk) before you start another speed interval. You've recovered when you are back to breathing a little harder than normal. Do this 3–5 times during each walk for 20–30 seconds each for at least 4 or 5 weeks, but don't do it every day. It's an every-other-day workout.

Experienced

Start timing yourself and measuring your heart rate (see page 166) during your walks.

ROWING MACHINE

Rowing Stats

Calories Burned*	Body-Shaping Potential
240–360 per half-hour	Tones the entire body, especially the muscles of the thighs, buttocks, abdominals, back and arms

*Based on a 10½ stone (67kg) woman. If you weigh more, you'll burn more calories; if you weigh less, you'll burn fewer.

Rowing indoors is a great way to whip your belly, butt and thighs into top-notch shape, particularly if your upper body yearns for something to do while you're working these areas. It's a great high-intensity workout that uses virtually all of your muscles in a flowing sequence. Because rowing isn't weight-bearing and therefore doesn't stress the leg joints, it's excellent for women with troublesome knees or weak ankles. (Outdoor rowing, if you can do it, burns nearly as many calories as cross-country skiing.)

Body-Shaping Benefits

Here's what to expect when you use your rowing machine regularly.

- You'll burn calories galore, because you're using all four limbs while your heart works – which burns more calories than lower-body exercise alone.

- You contract your abdominal muscles when you're rowing so they become strong and toned. Your legs and butt do a tremendous amount of work, so they grow lean and strong too.

- As a bonus you'll tone and strengthen your upper arms, an added trouble spot for many women as they reach midlife.

Psychological Benefits

Rowing leaves you with more energy and generates endorphins, brain chemicals that cause relaxation and euphoria. If you're a loner, rowing lets you work out in your own time, at your own pace, at home or in a gym. But if you enjoy being with others and crave competition, look for an indoor rowing class (where everyone in the class rows her own machine, but the instructor plays group leader).

The Right Gear

Shoes and clothes. Wear low-cut trainers to allow a range of motion in your ankles. Loose clothes, such as T-shirts, can get caught in the machine and won't allow you to move as smoothly, so wear an exercise top and something close-fitting such as cycling shorts.

The right machine. You may already have an indoor rower. If so, check that it has not become creaky or damaged over the years. If so, it may need a little oil to return to working order.

But, unless your shoulders are very strong, you may be better off not using an older machine at all. Many machines made in the 1980s feature two 'oars' that move independently of one another (rather than a pulley), along with piston-driven resistance. Both features can make rowing potentially stressful on the shoulders.

Here's what to look for.

- *Sturdy equipment with an ample seat and adjustable foot pads.* The only parts of your body that touch the rower are your hands, feet and backside. The foot pads should be easy to adjust for foot size. And when you row, the equipment should remain steady and secure on the floor.

If you're big-bottomed, make sure you fit comfortably in the seat. Also, a big tummy may interfere with your range of motion and force you to hold your legs out to your sides, putting stress on the ligaments of your knees. Or you may round your back while rowing, which could lead to back problems. If you are very overweight, you may have to lose some by other means before you can start rowing. Or you could consider starting on a recumbent (see page 174).

■ *Air or water resistance.* Both air and water resistance give a smoother ride than the older piston-resistance machines, and they more closely simulate outdoor rowing.

■ *Space.* Rowing machines are long – at least 6ft (2m). So if you're buying, make sure you have enough room for it.

Getting Started

Done properly, rowing is a fluid, full-body motion. Your hands grasp the bar with an overhand grip while your feet are in foot pads and your butt is in a seat. The seat glides along a track as your legs flex and extend. Your arms rhythmically straighten and bend as you propel yourself through the rowing motion. That said, rowing looks easier than it is. Even with the seat properly adjusted, it requires good posture and a lot of flexibility.

Warm up. To avoid stress to your muscles or knees warm up for a few minutes (a treadmill or exercise bike are ideal) and make sure that your knees do not bend to an angle less than 90 degrees. Stretch your leg muscles, especially your hamstrings and lower back, before you get on your machine.

As you begin to row, move backwards. Your arms should be at a 90-degree angle with your body, and your shoulder blades should move backwards and towards each other. As you glide forwards, your arms should straighten as far as the rope or chain will allow. Take time to row properly. And if you have lower-back problems, get some rowing tuition in a gym before you begin your exercise programme.

Here's a step-by-step guide.

The catch. This is the first movement of the series and begins with you sitting close to the front of the machine. Your hands hold the bar, your arms are straight and you are leaning slightly forward. Your knees are bent at a 90-degree angle, with your shins perpendicular to the floor.

The drive. With this motion, you begin to go backwards. Your legs straighten, and as your hands pass above your knees your torso begins to move back and your arms to bend.

Tips for Rowers

• Many rowing machines come with a digital readout of distance travelled, time elapsed and calories used, so that you can track your progress and intensity level. Heart rate monitors are also available with some models. Machines can also be programmed to time your rest and work time if you want to do interval training.

• When you start, don't try to go as fast as possible. You'll tire out too quickly and not burn as much fat as you want. Instead, warm up on an exercise bike, then move to the rowing machine and go at a moderate pace for about 20 minutes. Going longer, rather than fast, will burn more fat.

• Once you get used to the machine, try to increase your intensity for 30 seconds at a time, then slow down for 30 seconds. At first you'll be able to do so for only 20 minutes (if that), but eventually you will work your way up to a longer workout of 40 minutes or so. Be sure to warm up for 5 minutes and stretch your hamstrings and lower back first. Cool down for 5–10 minutes after rowing. Once your heart rate drops below 90 beats per minute, it is safe for you to stop completely.

The finish. Bend your elbows and bring the bar towards your abdomen. (Straighten your legs without locking your knees.)

The recovery and preparation. To return to the catch and resume the pattern, stretch and straighten your arms and pivot on your hips. Now let your knees slowly come up and bend to a 90-degree angle as you glide back towards the front of the machine.

What *not* to do. With rowing, what you shouldn't do is as important as what you should do. Don't lock your knees or your elbows when you're at either end of the stroke. Although your legs and arms will be 'straight', you can protect your joints by keeping them loose, relaxed and slightly flexed.

Use your back and legs equally, rather than focusing on the pulling motion of your upper body. Your arms and legs should move in a rhythmic, flowing motion as part of the equipment.

Finally, don't give up: learning how to row properly takes a long time. In the beginning, you push yourself mentally because you have to learn proper form and technique. The physical challenge of a tough workout comes later.

Rowing Workouts

BEGINNER

Row for 20 minutes at least twice a week. Keep the resistance light, but not so light that momentum moves you.

INTERMEDIATE

Row hard for 30 seconds, then easy for 30 seconds. Try to do 20–40 minutes at least 3 times a week.

EXPERIENCED

If you are rowing at this advanced level, warm up for 5–10 minutes, then keep a steady, high-intensity pace going for 40–60 minutes. Don't bend your knees past a 90-degree angle. Cool down. Repeat 4 or 5 days a week.

SKIPPING

For the busy woman on a budget, skipping is the ultimate calorie-burning exercise. It doesn't take a lot of time, it's inexpensive and it's high-intensity.

Body-Shaping Benefits

The rewards include:

- You'll burn calories – lots of them. Skipping is on a par with running when it comes to calorie burn.
- You'll improve endurance, coordination, balance and timing.
- You'll strengthen your bones as well as your muscles; this is a great bonus, because it helps prevent osteoporosis.

The Right Gear

Shoes. Since you're going to be doing a lot of bouncing on the balls of your feet, wearing the right shoes is important. Otherwise you could sprain an ankle or tear a tendon. You'll need a quality pair of aerobic or cross-training shoes to give you cushioning and support in all the right places. When you're in the shop, jump up and down to make sure the shoes fit right.

Clothes. You probably know by now whether you're more comfortable in an exercise bra – but this is an activity where you might even want two. Women who take a bra size 36 or larger usually do best by layering two running bras on top of each other, and then wearing a close-fitting T-shirt or tank on top of that.

Rope. Once upon a time an old clothesline would have done. Now you have many more choices:

- *Spring for the swivel.* The rope should swivel within the handles or at the handles, so that it doesn't twist on itself while you're jumping.
- *Choose right.* Skipping ropes come in a range of materials. Starting out, you might choose a segmented rope (otherwise known as a beaded rope) or one made of woven cotton or synthetic material. The segmented ropes have a nylon cord at the centre that is strung with cylindrical plastic beads that look like hollow noodles. A woven rope, made of nylon, cotton or polypropylene, resembles the old-fashioned kind, and won't sting as much if you happen to swat your back.

  After you've advanced a bit, you might choose a speed rope or licorice rope. They're made from vinyl plastic, and they're light and fast. Leather ropes are just as fast as speed ropes, but wear out sooner. Some advanced jump skippers who are in very good physical condition choose weighted ropes that can weigh up to 6lb (3.8kg).

- *Measure for leisure.* When a rope is the right length you can hold it at waist-level and hardly move your hands, and it will clear your head and feet with no problem. (If you have to circle your arms around, the rope's too short; if it bounces and hits your ankles, it's too long.) To get a comfortable length, stand with one or both feet in the middle of the rope, then lift the handles as high as they'll go. If they reach your armpits, you have what you want. Some ropes are adjustable, and others can be shortened just by putting in a couple of overhand knots near the handles.

- *Find the space.* Even though it's convenient to

skip at home, it's sometimes hard to find enough room. If you're average height, you'll need at least a 9ft (3m) ceiling, with plenty of space around you. The lawn won't work because the rope gets tangled in the grass, and carpet slows you down. So you might head for the cellar, garage or patio. That's fine, as long as you're on a surface that has a little give to it, like wood or hard rubber. You don't want to jump on hard concrete or tile, which don't give any bounce and are murder on your joints.

■ *Go to the mat.* You can convert a thick carpet to a jump-friendly surface by using a plastic mat of the kind placed under an office desk or chair. These are available at larger office supply stores. To convert the floor in a garage or spare room into a jump-friendly surface, consider investing in plastic interlocking tiles, as used in indoor courts for sports such as volleyball and gymnastics. A hard rubber mat or flooring are good, too, but avoid squishy aerobics mats because they have too much give.

Jump . . . for Joy!

• **Enjoy!** Skipping can be intense – but with music in the background, and maybe some kids or friends to keep you company, it's fun too. Plus it travels well. Just pack your rope and shoes, and you can skip wherever you go.

• **Warm to the task.** Start out with an easy, two-footed jump. Wait a few minutes, until your muscles get warmed up, before you try jumping faster. After you feel comfortable and warm jumping with both feet, try a light jog step.

• **Alternate high- and low-impact jumping.** You can't expect to do high-impact jumping for half an hour, so you have to combine it with low-impact moves. When you stop to take a breather, try marching on the spot for a while.

• **Mix and match.** For a high-intensity interval workout combine skipping with circuit training. For instance, after a warm-up, you might alternate skipping with push-ups, triceps dips and squats. Or, combine rope work with cardiovascular activities such as walking briskly around the gym and riding an exercise bike. You can also use skipping as the high-intensity portion of a less intense, regular workout. For example, if you like to walk you can take your usual route, then return home

for a minute or two of skipping. This will raise your heart rate and increase the intensity of your routine.

• **Into the rhythm.** Once you get the general rhythm of jumping, jump for up to three minutes, then do three minutes of weight training or resistance work. You'll notice a big change in the shape of your lower body if you alternate lower-body routines with high-intensity skipping a couple of times a week.

• **Variations.** There are hundreds. Try the heel dig jump: with each jump you bring one leg in front of your body as if you were digging in your heel. It looks like a Cossack dance without the deep squat or the funny hat. If you're feeling more ambitious, you might try crossing your arms when you jump – though don't be surprised if you get tangled up at first. Or try jump-rope jacks, where you land with your feet apart on the first jump, then bring your feet together on the second jump.

• **Join others.** Skipping rope with others helps you beat boredom and stick with your routine. Many classes are held in conjunction with kick boxing or martial arts classes, and they're offered at aerobics studios. Local gyms, YWCAs, kick boxing schools, and martial arts schools are likely to have information. Just call and ask.

Getting Started

'If you're just starting out and haven't skipped rope in years, just ease into it.

Skip the skip. Begin jumping with both feet, but try to do it without that little skip between jumps. Jump just high enough to clear the rope, and bring the rope over fast so you don't have time for that extra hop. Start out at the easiest pace you can without having to add the hop.

Pedal your feet. For variation, try jogging from foot to foot as you jump. The motion is more like pedalling a bike or light jogging. You control the intensity by how fast you 'jog'

through your rope. Keep your posture as erect as possible.

Keep your elbows in and wrists relaxed. With your elbows tucked close by your sides, your arms should barely move while you're skipping. Swing the rope with a relaxed motion of your forearms and wrists.

Stick to the low-jump. Don't rise more than 1in (2.5cm) off the ground. The rope should just clear the space between your feet and the mat.

Stop when you want to. If you're tired after a minute or two of skipping, take a break – then try again when you feel like it.

Skipping Workouts

BEGINNER

5–20 minutes of easy 2-footed jumping, paying attention to form. Start out with five 1-minute sessions between other interval activities. Work up to doing 1-minute jumping intervals for half the time. Do this combination 3 or 4 times a week.

INTERMEDIATE

20–40 minutes of 2-footed jumping – or alternating between 1-footed and 2-footed jumping – 3 or 4 times a week. Jump for 2-minute intervals, broken up by 3 minutes of another activity, so you are jumping two-thirds of the time.

EXPERIENCED

Alternate 3 minutes of skipping with 3 minutes of other activities for a total of 40–60 minutes.

SPINNING

Spinning Stats

Calories Burned*	Body-Shaping Potential
About 535 per 45-minute class	Trims your butt and thighs, tones your abdominal muscles

*Based on a 10½ stone (67kg) woman. If you weigh more, you'll burn more calories; if you weigh less, you'll burn fewer.

Also known as studio cycling, spinning is basically road cycling brought indoors. It's done on a specially designed workout bike and is set to music or a series of visualisations.

Even if you have tried an exercise bike and hated it, you'll love spinning. For one thing, it simulates riding a real bike much better. A spinning bike has a weighted fly-wheel, which picks up speed when you pedal, so you feel as if you're actually going down (or up) hills or just riding along a country road. You can also stand on a spin bike in order to climb the 'hills' with more power (and thus change the muscles you're working in your legs). Finally, spinning is a group activity. An instructor leads your ride – sometimes using visualisation, sometimes utilising speedwork, and sometimes combining every move you can do making for some of the most intense workouts you are likely to experience.

Body-Shaping Benefits

Here's what you can expect when you spin regularly.

- You'll burn 600–800 calories an hour – about as much as rowing on a machine at race pace.
- You'll tone your entire lower body, especially your butt and the front of your thighs.
- If you do a lot of standing and sitting intervals (known as jumps), you'll strengthen your abdominal muscles.

Psychological Benefits

Spinning is a true mind–body experience. The instructor will choose from a variety of 'rides', each of which will add to your mental pleasure. Some lead their students on imaginary trips through the south of France, some lead you through intervals that simulate a road race, and others simply get you to close your eyes and stay in touch with the way your body feels as you pedal through a variety of intensities and positions.

The Right Gear

Footwear and clothes. As on traditional racing bikes, spinning bike pedals consist of a 'cage' to hold your foot steady, and a 'lock' for bike shoes. Locking your foot into the pedal helps you move your legs more smoothly, but not everyone likes the feel of bike shoes. Most bike pedal manufacturers have a universal lock, which means that most bike shoes will fit into any bike pedal, spinning or otherwise.

As with riding any bike, spinning can irritate sensitive spots. Cycling shorts have extra padding in the bottom and are available at most sports shops.

Water. Spinning bikes have built-in water-bottle holders because you need to stay hydrated during the class. Choose a bottle with a pop-up spout so you don't have to interrupt your ride to open up your bottle.

A towel. You'll need a small hand towel, not only to soak up sweat, but also to wipe down your bike before someone else uses it.

A gel seat. Some gyms provide bike seats filled with gel, while others expect you to bring your own. Gel seats have a lot more give than a traditional bike seat and some people prefer them to padded cycling shorts – especially if they don't look good in close-fitting shorts or can't find them in their size.

Getting Started

Yes, spinning is a tough aerobic and lower-body workout. It takes three to four weeks before you begin to notice a build-up in the muscles and connective tissues in your legs. Start slowly and progress gradually.

Take a beginners' class. Most gyms offer one of these. The instructor will show you how to adjust your bike so that you're safe and comfortable as you ride. If the seat is too low or the pedal tension too high, for example, you may experience knee pain.

The five basic spinning moves are:

- *Seated flat.* The basic sitting position, used for warm-up, cool-down and speedwork.

- *Seated hill.* This is much the same position, but when you increase the resistance of the fly-wheel your butt will slide back to give your legs more power to pedal. Try to keep your upper body relaxed and, most important, don't jam the pedals on the downstroke. Your leg motion should remain fluid.

- *Standing hill.* Once the resistance forces you to incorporate more leg power, you'll want to stand up. Your pedalling will slow down, but your legs will work very hard and you'll feel the resistance of the bike. This will really work the muscles of your legs and butt.

- *Running.* In a standing position, you'll decrease the resistance on the fly-wheel, move your legs and torso slightly ahead of the seat and, with less resistance than you use when on a standing hill, push the pedals as quickly as possible without losing control. Spinners usually 'run' after a good warm-up to increase their heart rate and get to the next level of exertion.

- *Jumping.* Keeping the bike at a fairly high and consistent resistance level, you'll do some interval work. Without changing your pedalling rhythm you'll stand up for a measured amount of time, then sit down for the same time. Make sure you're not throwing your weight forward or pushing your legs down hard.

Vary your hand positions. Since spinning simulates road riding, your hand positions will vary depending on the ride.

- *Close together.* Used when you're seated, in this position your hands are next to each other, not grasping the handlebars too tightly. Your elbows and shoulders are always relaxed, with your knuckles slightly higher than your wrists. Your elbows should flare out a little.

- *Wider apart.* Used for seated climbing and jumping, in this position your hands are slightly separated and relaxed. Don't hold the handlebars too tightly.

- *On the ends of the handlebars.* Used only for standing climbing, in this position your hands are at the outer edges of the handlebars, with your knuckles facing out and your fingers wrapped around the bar.

Aim for balance between speed (how fast you pedal) and resistance (how hard it is to pedal). You want to keep some resistance on the fly-wheel or it will feel as if your legs are moving out of control.

Ride for yourself. There is no competition. No one can tell at what resistance level you're riding and no one will force you to stand when everyone else is standing or to jump if everyone else is jumping.

Spinning Workouts

BEGINNER

Take twice-weekly classes, with no jumping for 4–6 weeks.

INTERMEDIATE

Move on to 3 classes per week. To work your legs, work out at a slightly higher pedalling speed.

EXPERIENCED

After 2–3 months of steady riding (3 times a week), you're ready for the big time. Include jumping and other intense moves like sprinting (high-speed pedalling at light to moderate resistance, as if you're hurrying to finish a race).

STEP AEROBICS

Step Aerobics Stats

Calories Burned*	Body-Shaping Potential
Approximately 300 per half-hour using a 6in (15cm) step	Works the entire lower body – hips, thighs and buttocks

*Based on a 10½ stone (6/kg) woman. If you weigh more, you'll burn more calories; if you weigh less, you'll burn fewer.

A high-intensity, low-impact movement, step aerobics was born in the late 1980s. During a workout, you'll step on, over and around a bench, all in time to heart-pumping music. You don't have to be highly coordinated and you don't have to go to a gym. You can buy a step bench and videos from sports shops and catalogues, making step aerobics one of the least expensive and most effective home workouts.

Body-Shaping Benefits

Here's what you can expect when you do step aerobics regularly.

- You will burn lots of fat.
- You'll tone and shape the muscles in your lower body, especially your butt, thighs and calves.
- If you keep your abdominals contracted, you'll tone and strengthen those muscles.

Psychological Benefits

Step aerobics will improve your mood as well as your ability to think creatively. As a bonus, it can also help women who feel clumsy where choreography or footwork are concerned.

The Right Gear

Shoes. You'll want support so a good pair of aerobic shoes is your best bet. Look for flexible ones with plenty of cushioning and arch support. Some women prefer higher-cut shoes that give their ankles extra support.

Step bench. This is basically a low, wide platform with graduated risers, so you can increase step height as you become more experienced. Some risers are attached to the step and simply fold under it when you want to change the height.

Here's what to look for:

- *Sturdy construction* The bench should feel as solid as any step you would climb in your house. Likewise, any risers should be solid and not wobble as you go up and down the bench.
- *A step that is wide and long enough* You need plenty of room for both your feet on the bench. Some choreography won't work with a narrow step. You should also be able to take at least one step out to the side while you're on the bench. The ideal step is 2ft (60cm) wide and 3ft (1m) long. You can buy shorter (and cheaper) step benches, but the longer and wider the bench, the more intense your workouts.

Getting Started

Step is a high-intensity exercise, so begin your workout slowly. Experts recommend videos specifically geared towards beginners. Here's how to use them:

Take baby steps. The basic step pattern goes 'up-up, down-down' – up with the right foot, up with the left foot, down with the right foot, down with the left foot. Remember to place your whole foot on the step, not just your toes or the ball of your foot.

At first you'll have to look to make sure your foot is in the right position. Eventually you'll get a feel for it, and you can look ahead, not down, and follow the tape or instructor.

First master the legs, then add your arms. Concentrate on getting the foot patterns down and feeling comfortable using the platform. When you're ready, begin to incorporate arm movements. Continuous arm movements increase your heart rate, and thus the number of calories you burn, by up to 10 per cent.

Forget the hand weights. Hand weights can limit movement and can cause pain and fatigue in your shoulders when used for long periods.

Limit yourself to four step workouts a week. Studies have shown that doing step aerobics more than four times a week markedly increases the risk of injury. So be happy that it's a high-intensity workout that will burn lots of calories in a very short time.

Increase step height very gradually. The Reebok stepping platform – considered a 'benchmark'-size step by experts – is 6in (15cm) high. You can adjust the height by 2in (1 cm) at a time to make the advanced step bench a total height of up to 10in (25cm).

When you feel comfortable doing your step routine at the lowest height, add height 2in (1cm) at a time until your leg reaches a 60-degree angle or a comfortable step height. Only very tall or extremely advanced exercisers should use a step bench higher than 10in (25cm). Step height (combined with your body weight) is the biggest variable in terms of how many calories you'll burn.

How Beth Burned Off Pounds and Years with Step Aerobics

When 41-year-old mother of three Beth went to a restaurant with some friends they passed through the bar, which was packed with men. 'But none of them looked at me at all,' she says. 'I was 35 at the time, but I looked a lot older.'

At 5ft 1in (1.5m) and 10 stone (63.6kg), Beth decided to do something. 'I had always been put off aerobics classes because everyone would look better than me ,' she says. 'But I thought I'd be all right exercising in my own home. So I went to the library and borrowed some tapes. But I still didn't like aerobics.'

Then someone lent Beth a step bench and step aerobics tape and she loved it. 'It was easy for me to build my confidence. For some reason – because the music is slower – my feet and brain work better with step than with aerobics.'

Beth started with a beginner's tape and then went on to increasingly advanced ones. 'I've found that I'm always able to pick up the choreography after using one tape just a few times,' she says. 'When I get a new tape I really have to concentrate at first. As I become more comfortable with it, I'm able to focus more on giving my body a tough workout. I do some of my best thinking when I'm using some of the tapes I'm most comfortable with.'

Step aerobics has really paid off for Beth. She now weighs about 8 stone 2lb (52.2kg). 'My thighs are slimmer, firmer and much more muscular,' she notes. 'But more than that, I don't look my age.'

Step Aerobics Workouts

BEGINNER

Perform a 30-minute workout that begins with an 8-minute warm-up and ends with a 5-minute cool-down. Start by doing this twice a week for 3 weeks to 1 month.

INTERMEDIATE

Increase one of 3 things: intensity (use harder moves and/or more arm combinations); duration (work out for a total of 40–50 minutes); or the number of times you exercise (try 3 or 4 times a week). Don't increase all at once, and keep switching things around for 4–6 weeks.

EXPERIENCED

Add the hard moves, like lunges. Don't work out for longer than 60 minutes, or more often than 4 times per week.

STEPPING AND STAIRCLIMBING MACHINES

Stepping and Stairclimbing Stats

Calories Burned*	Body-Shaping Potential
250–350 calories per half-hour	Tones butt, thighs, hips and calves

*Based on a 10½ stone (67kg) woman. If you weigh more, you'll burn more calories; if you weigh less, you'll burn fewer.

Are you intimidated by – yet envious of – those slender women moving up and down on the long line of stairclimbing machines at the gym? Well, there's a good reason these women are so svelte. Few workouts trim and tone your butt and thighs as efficiently as stepping. The key to being consistent is finding an effective form of distraction. On a step machine you can read, watch television, listen to music or programme the machine to vary your workouts.

Although the terms *stepper* and *stairclimber* are used interchangeably, they are different machines. Steppers work only your lower body. You balance on the handlebars, pushing with one foot at a time, alternately. Climbers work the whole body.

Body-Shaping Benefits

Repeatedly raising and lowering your body with either a stepper or stairclimber uses all of the large muscles in your hips, butt, thighs and lower legs. As a result, stepping combines calorie burning with lower-body sculpting.

Here's what you can expect when you use a stepper regularly:

- You'll tone and strengthen your butt and thigh muscles, leaving you with a smaller butt and leaner thighs.
- You'll develop shapelier calf muscles.

The Right Gear

Shoes. Any type of athletic shoe or comfortable trainer will work on a step machine, so you don't have to buy elaborate footwear.

Beat the Monotony of Endless Climbing

Once you've been slogging up and down on a step machine for a while you will probably want a change in routine.

• **Take the stairs.** You've heard it a thousand times: use the steps and not the lift at work. That's the way to work stairclimbing into your busy day. You can also use the stairs for 10 minutes of exercise a few times a day but not in heels. They will throw you off balance and take a toll on your knees, especially when going down the stairs. Wear trainers, or at least flat heels.

• **Add your upper body.** If you like using a stepper but wish your upper body could get a workout, too, investigate vertical climbing machines. It's like climbing a stationary ladder, and because you work your arms and legs in a full range of motion you'll burn lots of calories.

Machines. You'll find steppers or stairclimbers in most gyms, so you don't have to buy one unless you want to. And good ones are expensive.

Here are some questions to ask and features to think about when you're considering a step machine at a gym or shopping for a home model.

- *Is it sturdy?* The equipment should support your weight easily and remain steady even while you're in motion. The pricier machines are sturdier and a better buy for people who have lots of weight to lose.

- *Is it the right size?* Every step machine has a prescribed range of distance that the foot pad can travel as you step. Some ranges are wider than others. It should be easy for you to stay in the midrange, or 'sweet spot', of the step length. Likewise, the foot pads should be big enough to hold your entire foot with room to spare.

- *How does it work?* There are two kinds of step machine, dependent and independent. If you push down on one step of a dependent machine the other step will rise, creating greater stress on the knee joint. Independent steps aren't connected by anything and involve more natural and less stressful movement.

Most makes of step machine offer display monitors with manual or programmed features that set and measure the time and intensity of your effort. The programmes also help you check your progress and guide you through a variety of workouts. But you don't need an elaborately programmed unit to get a good workout. Choose a machine based on how the equipment moves as you exercise, not on the display features.

- *What type of resistance does it use?* Experts recommend buying hydraulic, cable or chain steppers. Be careful, though, since hydraulic machines (which are cheaper) use oil, which can stain carpets.

Getting Started

Stepping might look easy, but doing it wrong can cost you 75 calories per workout and contribute to aches and pains during and afterwards. To step safely and effectively, you have to do it right.

Warm up. As with any exercise, start slow and stop gradually. Warm up for 5 minutes with smaller steps on low resistance, then move into your workout with longer steps at a higher resistance. Slow down again at the end, and make sure you stretch your leg muscles afterwards.

Don't lean on the rails. When people lean they do about 20–25 per cent less work than the machine credits them for, because they aren't using their full body weight. If you're working so hard that you have to lean on the machine, reduce the speed. Your hands should rest lightly, if at all, on the handlebars.

Slow down. Stepping quickly doesn't mean you'll burn more calories. It's the force of your leg working against the step, not how fast you step, that determines the value of the workout. Your steps should cover the middle range of the whole length of the step, and your speed should be steady.

Stepping Workouts

BEGINNER

5 minutes at the lowest level you feel comfortable with, every day if possible. Work your way up to 20 minutes at this intensity.

Intermediate

Once you can do 20 minutes of exercise every day, cut down on frequency but increase intensity. Exercise for 2 days on and 1 day off, raising the intensity level every few workouts. Aim for 20 minutes, 3 or 4 times per week.

Experienced

Alternate high and moderate intensity: for every minute of high-intensity exercise do 2 minutes of moderate intensity. Continue for 20 minutes, 3 or 4 times a week.

Swimming

Swimming Stats

Calories Burned*	Body-Shaping Potential
249–351 per half-hour, depending on what stroke you do and how fast you swim	High-calorie burning; tones the legs, hips, torso, arms, back and chest

*Based on a 10½ stone (67kg) woman. If you weigh more, you'll burn more calories; if you weigh less, you'll burn fewer.

Few activities are as sensual and relaxing as swimming. And swimming may be the perfect start for a woman who needs to lose a few pounds, because extra fat helps keep you buoyant, making it easier to swim better and faster.

Swimming isn't weight-bearing – it doesn't subject your joints and bones to a lot of impact. You're expending a lot of energy, which burns calories, but you don't have to support your body weight while you do it.

Body-Shaping Benefits

Here's what you can expect when you swim regularly:

- You'll burn as many calories as running, without stressing your knees or bones.
- You'll tone your abdomen and hips.
- You'll tone and strengthen your legs. As a bonus, you'll also firm up your chest and upper arms.

Psychological Benefits

Many women hate the idea of getting into a bathing suit but feel beautiful once they're actually in the water and their body seems so much lighter. If you're substantially overweight, having the weight of your body off your bones and joints for an hour or so may also be a physical relief and supply extra energy.

The Right Gear

Footwear. You could swim barefoot. But if you're swimming to shape up, experts recommend the following footwear:

- *Fins.* Available at shops that sell equipment for water sports, fins help you swim faster and give your legs a better workout. They create more resistance against the water for your muscles, so you kick faster. Go for medium-length fins, not extra-short. The length is what helps you go fast.

- *Shower sandals.* To protect yourself against the fungal infection athlete's foot, wear rubber flip-flops or sandals to walk to the pool and when you take a shower.

A pool. Maybe you'll be swimming in a lake or the sea, or are lucky enough to have your own pool. But most women who swim regularly are probably doing lengths at their local public pool.

Bathing suit. If you swim for exercise, buy a racing suit from a sports shop. You're looking not for something to lounge in, but for something that will hold your body in place and keep you streamlined in the water. For large-breasted women, fitness swimsuits with support are available.

Goggles. To minimise levels of harmful bacteria pool water must contain a certain amount of chlorine and other disinfecting chemicals that can irritate your eyes, so you need goggles. They're a must for swimming lengths because they allow you to see the lane markers on the bottom of the pool. Goggles aren't expensive; go to a sports shop and choose the best-fitting ones. Beginners need goggles with good peripheral vision and padding

Gigi Lost It in the Pool

When Gigi, 39, heard that she had raised cholesterol she couldn't deny she had a problem: she weighed 22 stone (140kg).

Ironically, when she got the phone call from the doctor she was eating chicken and chips and had a bowl of rich, vanilla ice cream waiting in the fridge. Soon afterwards, she started a low-fat, low-cal way of eating. 'I didn't starve myself. I still ate three whole meals daily, which totalled about 1200 calories.'

At about the same time that Gigi started to eat better, a swimming club opened up nearby. Remembering how she had loved to swim as a child, she began to swim five days a week and sometimes six in the hot days of summer. 'The weight just rolled off me,' she says. 'By July, I needed to tie a cord around my shorts to keep them up.'

Less than a year after starting to swim regularly, Gigi was 11 stone 6lb (72.7kg) lighter.

So how did Gigi manage to get her bathing suit on and step into the pool when so many thinner women feel too self-conscious to swim? 'I focus on my swimming goals, not on my weight,' she says. 'Plus, it's not as intimidating as you might think. In a pool, you see what real women look like and that makes it easier.'

Gigi believes that two key things have led to her successful weight loss. First, she chose an activity she loves. 'Whenever I make plans, my first priority is to work out when I can get my swim in,' she says.

Second, 'I was willing to let go of my old habits in order to make way for new, healthier ones. I was open to different foods and a new way of life. When you start seeing results and your plan comes together, it makes everything worthwhile.'

---

around the rim of the eyepiece. You should feel light suction around the eyes – just enough to keep water out.

Bathing cap. Public pools sometimes require women (and sometimes men) to wear a cap. It also helps protect your hair from chemicals, which can dry or discolour your hair. And if your hair is long, a cap keeps it from becoming tangled while you swim. Look for something sleek and simple: a silicone bathing cap is best because it doesn't pull your hair as much as other materials do.

Getting Started

Swimming for exercise is not the same as taking a dip when you want to cool off. You must swim at a consistent pace for at least 20 minutes to get your heart pumping and your fat burning.

Crawl first. Unless you're proficient at another stroke (breast, back, side or butterfly), you'll probably want to do the crawl, which is

Swimming Workouts

BEGINNER

Swim freestyle lengths for a total of about 100–300yd/ 90–250m every other day or at least 3 times a week for 1–2 months. If you have to stop between lengths at first, that's OK. Work up to swimming non-stop for 10 minutes. If you use fins, you'll burn more calories.

INTERMEDIATE

Swim 350–550yd/300–500m in about 15 minutes without stopping, at least 3 times a week for 2 months.

EXPERIENCED

Swim 600yd/550m (24 lengths in a 25yd/23m pool) to 880yd/ 800m at a time without stopping, 3 times a week. Mix and match your strokes, if you want. This should take about 30 minutes.

sometimes called freestyle swimming. Before you attempt to learn other strokes, work towards doing the crawl for 10 minutes at a time.

Warm up and cool down. Don't forget to warm up before swimming and cool down afterwards. Do at least 5 minutes of water exercise and stretching before you begin to swim lengths. To warm up, walk in the shallow part of the pool or tread water. To cool down, do the stretches in Stretch into Shape in chapter 10. Stay in the shallow end of the pool and use the steps or edge of the pool if you need to hold on to something.

Learn to roll. The real source of a swimmer's power comes from the hips and trunk. The key is to move from your hips, turning your head to one side to breathe as the opposite arm comes out of the water, then starting to roll towards the other side for your next breath and its matching stroke.

Turn your head and breathe in. Turn your whole head along with your body to one side and your mouth will lift slightly out of the water for an inhalation. As your body rolls back into a straight line, you'll slowly blow bubbles as you exhale into the water. Continue your body roll to the other side, turning your mouth out of the water on the other side for your next inhalation. Alternating breathing in this way helps to balance your stroke. When you become a proficient swimmer, alternate breathing sides every third pull.

Lead with your head. Your head, not your chin, should lead the way down the lane. You want your body in a streamlined position so that you're looking towards the floor of the pool. Don't worry about hitting the wall – when you see the end of the black line in your lane, start to make your turn.

Watch out for other swimmers. Chances are you'll be sharing the pool with others, so you have to learn your pool's lane-sharing etiquette. Check for notices before you enter the water.

Power Up in the Pool

You'll burn more calories if you go beyond the basic crawl and add other strokes to your repertoire

• **Flip on to your back.** A major calorie burner (345 calories per half-hour if you weigh 10½ stone/67kg), the backstroke is a wonderful complement to the crawl. If you don't like to keep your face in the water, you'll like this stroke.

• **Stay on your side.** This stroke doesn't burn the most calories (249 per half-hour if you weigh 10½ stone/67kg), but it's a relaxing way to cool down and work the oblique muscles along your torso. Toned obliques mean a toned waistline.

• **Fly like a butterfly.** Toughest to master, the butterfly pays off in terms of calories burned (351 per half-hour if you weigh 10½ stone/67kg).

• **Learn the new breast stroke.** The breast stroke has been reinvented and now calls for more whip in the kick and a more efficient, faster, narrower arm motion that doesn't strain your muscles as much as the old method, which required a complete extension of the arms. The breast stroke is also harder than it used to be. But it's still a great way to strengthen your pectoral muscles (and thus lift your breasts). You'll burn 330 calories per half-hour if you weigh 10½ stone (67kg).

TENNIS

Tennis Stats

Calories Burned*	Body-Shaping Potential
Burns 475 calories an hour in a highly competitive match	Tones the gluteus, quadriceps, hamstring and calf muscles

*Based on a 10½ stone (67kg) woman. If you weigh more, you'll burn more calories; if you weigh less, you'll burn fewer.

Chris Evert, Martina Hingis, the Williams sisters – great players, all. You don't have to play like a pro, however, to develop a body about which you can crow. If you normally get no closer to a tennis court than the television screen during Wimbledon fortnight, think again.

Body-Shaping Benefits

Whichever arm you use primarily to play tennis will become stronger and shapelier as a result of playing the game, but this sport primarily provides a lower-body workout. If you play regularly:

- Your gluteus (in your backside), quadriceps (along the front of your thighs), hamstrings (back of your thighs) and calf muscles will all get a good workout from the quick starts and stops and lateral movements required in tennis.

The Right Gear

Shoes. Running shoes are not designed for the game's constant lateral movement. If you wear proper tennis shoes, you'll run less risk of ankle injury. Here's what to look for:

- *Good arch support.* A shoe that's well designed for racket sports will have good support for the arch and be well-padded at the ball of the

foot, where you exert the most pressure. If the arch supports feel too high, try another style.

- *Toe room.* There should be just enough room in the toebox to move your toes and avoid blisters. That means no more than ¼in (6mm) between the toes and the toebox or front of the shoe. The toebox is subject to the most wear and tear during tennis, so make sure it's made of leather or rubber, not fabric, which will wear out faster.

- *Wide soles.* The sole should be wider than the upper, otherwise you won't be getting enough lateral support as you move from side to side on the court. Look for a midsole made of ethyl vinyl acetate (EVA) or polyurethane. Some shoes have air or gel within the midsole. Press the shoe. The midsole should give a bit. The insole should be made of fabric that will breathe and control moisture.

- *The right size.* Buy tennis shoes half a size larger than your regular shoe size, so they can accommodate tennis socks.

- *Socks.* Look for thick socks in moisture-wicking fabric or synthetic/cotton blends that provide extra cushioning to absorb shocks and prevent blisters. Ankle-length socks are best. Some players wear two pairs of socks to minimise blisters and maximise moisture absorption and cushioning.

Clothes. Some tennis clubs have a dress code requiring women to wear a skirt or a dress and men to wear a collared shirt. Others permit you to wear shorts. Some allow only all white attire, or light colours. Of course, if you're playing on a public court you can wear what you please.

Whatever you wear should be comfortable, but not baggy or too snug. If you wear clothing that's too large, the excess fabric may slow you down. Clothing that's too tight can restrict your movements and not allow your skin to breathe. If you wear shorts instead of a tennis skirt, look for wide legs and side vents to give you freedom of movement. Wear a sports bra to control bounce.

Cotton fabric is traditional for tennis, but it's best when blended with synthetics like Lycra, which help clothing keep its shape longer and resist wrinkling.

The right racket. Beginners should buy a lightweight, oversize racket, which will improve their chances of making contact with the ball. If your racket's too heavy your arm will get tired. But if it's too light you'll be waving it like a wand, not learning proper strokes.

Look for a racket with mid-level string tension, to absorb impact but provide power. As for grip, a finger's width should separate the tip of your middle finger from the crease at the base of your thumb as you grasp the handle.

Fresh balls. All tennis balls are created equal, so if you can buy a can cheaper at a discount store, do so. However, balls last longer in warmer climates.

Getting Started

Take lessons. Private tennis lessons can be expensive. Check at your local community centre or public library for more affordable tennis clinics and workshops.

Don't commit to a series of lessons (or a club membership) until you've taken at least one lesson. That way, you can see if you like the tennis pro and the game itself.

Choose your court. Grass is a difficult surface on which to learn tennis; hard surfaces are better. But if you're just starting out, look for an indoor court. There will be no sun to

blind you, no wind to skew your shots and a less distracting background that enables you to see the ball better.

Warm up. You're not going to get a tennis workout if you have to sit on the sidelines with a pulled muscle, so warm up before you play. Start with brisk walking or easy jogging, then stretch for several minutes. Calf muscles in particular can get tight, so stretch your quadriceps and hamstrings before, between and after games.

The intensity of any workout depends on whether the games include much rallying. So if you are scoring lots of quick points you may want to extend the time you play.

Conversely, if you plan to play for an hour but your racket feels like a lead weight after 45 minutes, listen to your body. Otherwise, you'll ache next day.

Tennis Workouts

BEGINNER

Enjoy non-competitive play for at least half an hour against someone of equal or greater ability.

INTERMEDIATE

Play competitively for 45 minutes to an hour.

EXPERIENCED

Engage in an hour to 90 minutes of tournament-type play.

WALKING

Walking Stats

Calories Burned*	Body-Shaping Potential
100 per mile	Tones abdominals, hips, thighs and buttocks

*Based on a 10½ stone (67kg) woman. If you weigh more, you'll burn more calories; if you weigh less, you'll burn fewer.

What could be simpler than putting one foot in front of the other? You don't need any fancy equipment and it can give you all the rewards of aerobic exercise, while putting less stress on your knees, hips and back. It can help lower your risk of heart disease, reduce your cholesterol and blood pressure, speed up fat loss and increase muscle tone.

Body-Shaping Benefits

Here's what you can expect when you walk regularly:

- Your body will burn more calories and more fat all day long because you've revved up your metabolism.
- You'll help tone your abdominals, hips, thighs and buttocks.
- You'll use all the major muscles – glutes, quads, hamstrings, back, biceps and triceps

Psychological Benefits

Walking makes you feel better. Cynthia Gates Baber, a social worker and psychotherapist in Atlanta, conducted a study of 25 women taking a race-walking class. At the start of the eight-week programme, Baber discovered that 48 per cent of the women showed signs of stress, and almost half had been in therapy for depression. By the end, only 32 per cent were still showing signs of stress.

The Right Gear

Shoes. Priority one for all walkers is good shoes. Look for:

- *Flexibility.* The shoe should bend where your foot bends – at the ball of your foot, not in the middle of the shoe.
- *An ample toebox.* When you walk, you bend and push off with your toes. There should be a thumb's width between the end of your longest toe and the front end of the shoe. If the toebox isn't big enough, your toes will be tingling 20 minutes into your walk.
- *Light, thin materials.* Look for shoes that are lightweight, with a thin heel and a flexible sole. Running and walking shoes with thick, cushioned soles are not good for walking. Also stay away from aerobics and tennis shoes.

Wet-weather gear. There's plenty of rain gear available to make wet-weather walking enjoyable.

Cold-weather gear. When it's cold outside, you want clothing in a fabric that pulls the moisture away from your skin. Look for T-shirts, turtlenecks and other garments in synthetic fibres designed for activewear. You can dress in layers, but don't wear cotton next to your skin because it won't wick away the sweat. Cover your ears, but even in cool weather, a hat may make your head perspire, so a headband is a better choice then. When the temperature dips below freezing, however, do wear a hat. If the weather is cool, wear gloves and when it gets really cold switch to mittens. Polar fleece is good for headbands and mittens because it doesn't trap moisture.

What Else You'll Need

Water. Drink 2 glasses of water about two hours before you walk, then one glass every 15–20 minutes during exercise. Afterwards, drink

Customise Your Walking Technique

- **Take short, quick steps instead of long strides.** You'll work your glute muscles in your buttocks.

- **Practise the heel-toe roll.** Push off from your heel, roll through the outside of your foot, then push through your big toe. Think of your big toe as the Go button and push off with propulsion. Keep your other toes relaxed. (This takes practice.)

- **Squeeze your glutes.** Imagine squeezing and lifting your glutes up and back, as if you were holding a £20 note between them. This will strengthen and tone those muscles. Developing the ability to maintain this deep contraction throughout your walk will take a while.

- **'Zip up' your abs.** During your walk, imagine you're zipping up a tight pair of jeans. Stand tall and pull your abdominal muscles up and in. You can practise this even when you're not walking. This will also strengthen your lower-back muscles.

- **Pump your arms.** Imagine that you're holding the rubber grips of ski poles in your hands. Stand straight, drop your shoulders, squeeze your shoulder blades behind you, and push your elbows back with each step. Keep your arm movements smooth and strong, moving past the outside of your hips.

- **Keep your chest up and shoulders back.** Use your walk as an opportunity to practise perfect posture. Imagine that someone has dropped ice down your back. That's the feeling you want to have as you hold your chest up and shoulders back.

- **Hold your head up.** Look about 10ft (3m) ahead of you. Imagine that you're wearing a baseball cap with the bill of the visor level to the horizon, so that you have to look up just enough to see the road. This keeps your neck aligned properly.

- **Smile and have fun.** Learning these techniques takes time and concentration. Be patient and enjoy your workouts. Dress comfortably; find a partner or wear headphones (if you're walking indoors only) and listen to music you love; and if you're walking outdoors, vary your route.

- **Practise mental fitness.** Don't replay the problems of the day while you walk. Try to maintain a state of relaxed awareness by paying attention to your breathing and noticing how your body feels. Visualise and tell yourself you're getting healthier, stronger and leaner.

1 pint (440ml) for each pound (0.5kg) of weight lost during the workout.

Sun protection. Wear sunscreen and a floppy, wide-brimmed hat or baseball cap, plus sunglasses with 100 per cent UV protection or a visor to shade your eyes and protect your face from sunburn. A visor is best for really hot weather because it doesn't hold the heat in.

Getting Started

Take it slow. If you need to lose 3½ stone (23kg) or are relatively inactive, don't overdo it at first. Aim for a daily 20-minute walk at a pace that makes your breathing just a bit laboured but doesn't leave you out of breath.

Keep going. If you can, walk the whole 20 minutes without stopping. But even if you can walk only 10 minutes at a time, you'll get some benefits. Slow down and rest for a few minutes, then begin again.

Listen to your heart. The best indicator of whether you're walking briskly enough to gain health benefits is your target heart rate.

Plan to walk every day. Even on days when you don't feel like doing it, just get outside and walk a short distance.

If you're an indoor walker, consider buying a treadmill, ideally a motorised version. Set it at a speed that lets you walk comfortably without holding on. When you feel balanced and are used to it, you can increase the speed. Walk on a treadmill for the same amount of time that you would if you were walking outside.

Walking Workouts

BEGINNER

20 minutes, 6 or 7 days a week for 2 weeks.

INTERMEDIATE

25 minutes, 6 or 7 days a week; increase walking time by 10 per cent increments each week until you reach 40 minutes.

EXPERIENCED

Continue to increase walking time by 10 per cent until you reach 45–60 minutes, 6 or 7 days a week. If you don't need to lose body fat you can walk 20–30 minutes, 3 days a week, to stay fit.

WATER AEROBICS

Water Aerobics Stats

Calories Burned*	Body-Shaping Potential
200–250 per half-hour	Tones abdominals, hips, thighs, buttocks, calves, arms and more

*Based on a 10½ stone (67kg) woman. If you weigh more, you'll burn more calories; if you weigh less, you'll burn fewer.

You don't have to know how to swim to do water aerobics (aquatics). As long as you're comfortable in water up to your chest, you're a candidate for this extraordinarily effective form of exercise. It's easy on your joints and still provides a great aerobic workout. The resistance provided by moving through water, which is 12 to 14 times greater than travelling over land, gives your muscles continuous resistance training.

Body-Shaping Benefits

Water workouts on a regular basis can bring you a steady stream of rewards.

- You'll burn calories just as well as if you did an aerobic workout on land, without the added stress on your joints.

- The three-dimensional effects of water provide resistance in all directions, toning your muscles from head to toe and creating a beautifully shaped and balanced body.

- You'll work your abdominal and back muscles, along with your legs, extra hard in the water to maintain erect body alignment and balance, resulting in strong, defined abdominals and legs.

Psychological Benefits

Water aerobics gives you a wonderful sense of well-being during and after a workout. The water offers a comfortable environment, and its massaging effects soothe tired muscles.

The Right Gear

Shoes. Water fitness shoes are soft and flexible and specifically designed for walking in water. They add comfort, have a nonskid base and help protect your feet. Water fitness trainers, which provide more support, are also a choice but, if you like, you can do water aerobics in bare feet.

Pool. The water should be approximately chest deep, and you should have enough space to move through a full range of motion without bumping into the side of the pool or the person next to you. The water temperature should be between 80°–85°F (27°–29°C). As your body temperature rises from the vigorous parts of the routine, this temperature keeps you cool.

Swimsuit. Comfort is the key here. Wear a suit that you can move well in. If you feel embarrassed because you're out of shape, just pull a T-shirt over your costume.

Resistance-training aids. Working out in the water tones your abs and helps to flatten your stomach. Adding other equipment, such as water dumbbells, polystyrene woggles and webbed gloves helps tone other muscle groups – notably your thighs, buttocks and arms – while increasing the intensity of your workout.

Flotation belt. For deep-water workouts a flotation belt is essential for safety and also provides good back support.

Getting Started

Instruction. Get a book or video, or investigate classes in your area (ask at your local swimming pool or library). A good class should include a warm-up, a gradually intensifying aerobics portion, muscle conditioning exercises and a cool-down consisting of flexibility exercises.

Tips for More Effective Water Workouts

• **Add variety.** Don't just do water walking and leave it at that. There's a huge range of things you can do, from length swimming to water yoga. Experiment with new things to sustain your interest.

• **Take a partner.** Working out with someone else keeps you committed and, once you're there, staying in the water longer and working out harder.

• **Keep a workout journal.** A record of what you've accomplished heightens your motivation. Include the date, how long you stayed in the water, the type of workout, any resistance training equipment you used, and the number of repetitions you did. Also jot down how you felt before, during and after your workout and any ideas for future workouts.

• **Watch a video before you work out.** Watching even a few minutes of a water aerobics video before you work out, whether you're on your own or in a class, teaches you something new about form or motivates you to exercise better.

• **Add music.** If you're working out on your own, add music to boost your energy level and make the workout more fun.

• **Try these techniques to add to the intensity:** lift your knees higher while water walking and take longer strides; jog or run instead of walking; cup your hands and push or pull the water away from you; add equipment that increases intensity, such as drag, buoyant or weighted equipment.

Warm up. Experts recommend that you perform a three- to five-minute warm-up in the water before a water aerobics workout. Start with knee lifts and then use straight leg kicks to warm your muscles. You may also want to stretch for 3–5 minutes before you get into the water.

Get your heart pumping. The aerobic portion of your workout can include anything from water walking to length swimming. Experts recommend that you gradually work up to your target heart rate and stay at that level for at least 20 minutes.

Cool down. Use the last 3–5 minutes of the aerobics segment of your workout to cool down. Gradually decrease the intensity, so your heart rate drops and you breathe more slowly.

Monitor your intensity. To get the most out of your workout and work at a safe level, keep track of how hard you're exerting yourself. Check your pulse is in your target heart rate zone (see page 166). If you can't comfortably hold a conversation with the person next to you, you're working too hard, she says.

Keep yourself nimble. Finish the class with the stretches you did to warm up. This will keep you flexible and prevent muscle soreness.

Get into the swim at least three to five times a week. If you're consistent, you'll reach your goals. Perform your water aerobics workout for at least 20 minutes, preferably on alternating days to allow for rest and recovery.

Water Aerobics Workouts

BEGINNER

Target heart rate 60–65 per cent of maximum, 2–3 days a week.

INTERMEDIATE

Target heart rate 65–75 per cent of maximum, 3–4 days a week.

EXPERIENCED

Target heart rate 75–90 per cent of maximum, 4–6 days a week.

PART FIVE

Self-Coaching the New You

Chapter 12

Your New
Food Attitude

The average woman trying to lose weight has lost 100lb (45.4kg), gained 125 (56.8), and been on 15 diets, says California dietitian Debra Waterhouse. So the chances are that you've tried to lose weight before, only to regain it.

The truth is, most people who lose weight and keep it off haven't done so by finding the perfect crash diet or sipping a magic drink that melts away their fat cells. Lifelong weight control focuses not on your belly, butt or thighs, but on your brain.

Women who lose weight and keep it off succeed because they change their eating habits and the way they regard food. They see their bodies and attitudes not as obstacles, but as vehicles to success. Further, they don't pin their hopes on a celebrity or other personality who will dictate an absolute path of what to eat and when. They rely on themselves.

How do you develop a new food attitude? By critically re-examining your attitudes and refocusing your energy on more effective strategies that put you in control.

Restyle Your Eating Style

Here are some common yet self-defeating mind-sets about food, along with some suggestions for changing them.

Old attitude: *all I have to do is tell myself not to eat so much.*
New attitude: *I'm going to make some changes where food is concerned: what I buy, where I store*

it, how I prepare meals, where I eat, what I do while I'm eating, and how I order at restaurants.

Cultivating a new food attitude means making meaningful decisions, not relying on willpower to avoid temptation, says Dr Kelly Brownell, director of the Yale University Center for Eating and Weight Disorders. He tells people to plan their meals, shop from a list, and go to the supermarket on a full stomach – time-honoured strategies that work.

If your fridge resembles a salad bar because you shopped wisely, you'll suffer only minor damage if your resolve weakens. But if you've filled the freezer with frozen pizza and double chocolate ice cream you're just storing up trouble for yourself.

Other suggestions include:

- Do nothing else while you eat.
- Eat at fixed times.
- Eat in one place.
- Don't clean up everything on your plate.

Old attitude: *the holidays are coming (or the office bash, a cousin's wedding or other food fest), so there's no point in even trying to watch what I eat right now.*
New attitude: *I'm going to develop coping strategies for tempting situations.*

'Don't make excuses, take control!' urges Dr Laurie L. Friedman of the Johns Hopkins Weight Management Center in Baltimore. Going to a party at someone's house? Offer to bring a salad, a low-calorie starter or some exotic fruit.

That way, you won't binge on cheesecake because you had no choice. If you do eat some cake, take a small portion and enjoy it. But never let yourself be at the mercy of food or the situation. At a buffet, walk through and look at everything before choosing. Just select a few things that are most appealing.

Old attitude: *starting today, I will never eat chocolate (or crisps, or cheeseburgers, or Danish pastries) again.*
New attitude: *I can still eat whatever I want – occasionally. I just need to set limits for myself and stick to them.*

Not every indulgence has to turn into a binge. Some women may have foods that they like a lot or that trigger a binge for them. 'While they're trying to lose weight,' says Dr Friedman, 'I ask them to avoid certain foods that might undermine their efforts. But vowing to avoid something for ever is an empty promise.' The long-term goal is moderation. For many people, high-fat foods lose appeal once they get used to eating healthier choices.

If you do have a craving for something fattening, pay extra attention to the taste and texture of each bite. Sometimes the idea or the smell is better than the taste. You may find that, after a bite or two, the pleasure fades and you can stop.

Old attitude: *well, of course I ate a carton of ice cream at the end of a perfectly healthy day of eating. I'm a slob, I have no self-control, and I deserve to look this way.*
New attitude: *no one is perfect. I'm going to think about why this happened, take steps to prevent it the next time, and give myself a break.*

Don't fall into the trap of telling yourself that you are either perfect, eating healthy foods in reasonable portions, or horrible, slipping up and eating a big piece of cake.

Instead, put your slip-up in perspective: over the course of a month, one 2000-calorie mistake won't make much difference. The real

danger lies in heaping guilt and despair on yourself because you're not perfect. If that happens, you'll probably react by eating even more.

Old attitude: *I'm just going to follow the high-protein, low-carbohydrate diet that worked for my boss. I know it's a fad, but she lost weight really fast.*
New attitude: *I need to identify my own food attitudes and plan strategies that work best for me*

The theory behind high-protein diets is that if the body doesn't have carbohydrates available, it will turn to stored fat for energy. A high-protein diet relies heavily on meat, eggs and other animal sources of protein, while minimising bread, potatoes and other carbohydrates.

This diet works in the short term because it controls calories, and you lose a lot of water weight. The problem is that you can't stay healthy on it for long. Animal foods are usually high in fat, and they don't provide enough vitamins and minerals or fibre. Also, when you restrict carbohydrates, your body breaks down lean muscle mass – exactly what you **don't** want to do to tone your muscles. Worse, your body can lapse into a dangerous state called ketosis, causing diarrhoea, headaches, weakness, low blood pressure, fatigue and sleeplessness. What's more, eating too much protein is hard on your kidneys.

So forget the high-protein diet – or any fad diet. Experts emphasise that any diet that eliminates certain food groups and depends heavily on others is unwise. It also does nothing to help you foster realistic eating patterns.

To do that, says Dr Brownell, 'evaluate your strengths and weaknesses and choose foods and cooking techniques that help you the most'.

Begin by keeping a food diary of everything you eat for a week. Count up the calories and divide by seven. Note the time you eat, what you are doing while you eat, and what you are feeling.

A food diary will help you identify 'automatic' eating habits, such as munching mindlessly when you're not hungry. You'll also be able to spot patterns that may be thwarting your efforts to lose weight. Do you skip meals, then overeat? Do you tend to eat higher-fat, higher-calorie foods after 10:00 p.m.? Once you know which situations are risky for you, you can either avoid them or plan how to deal with them. For instance, you might pack rice cakes as an afternoon pick-me-up at work, or decide not to eat in front of the television.

Keeping a food diary can even help keep you on track during the toughest times of the year – Christmas and other holidays.

Also, many people who maintain their weight loss continue monitoring their eating for a year or more. That way they see patterns over time, rather than dwelling on one bad day or one great week.

Old attitude: *I eat only salads, but I still gain weight. My problem is in my genes.*
New attitude: *weight control may be tougher for me than for other women, but I'm going to be honest with myself about what I eat.*

Most people eat much more than they think they do, recalling a 3oz (90g) steak when it was actually an 8oz (210g) steak, or forgetting the pastry they grabbed as they did some quick lunchtime shopping. When you keep a food diary, everything counts – even the chips you eat off your child's plate.

Grazing on junk food does make a difference if you are snacking several times a day. You also need to think about precisely what you're eating. A salad drenched in mayonnaise or oil-based dressing carries the same fat and calorie burden as cream sauce. Finally, consider whether you may have eaten an extremely low calorie diet for so long that you've slowed down your metabolism. Women who consistently eat fewer than 1200 calories a day burn fewer calories, so their attempts at losing weight go nowhere. You can get back to normal within a few months by eating at least 1200 calories a day and exercising to readjust your metabolism.

Old attitude: *I'm under a lot of stress now. I'll eat more sensibly when things calm down.*
New attitude: *things may never calm down. I have to find other ways to cope besides food.*

Stress is really just a euphemism for what psychologists see as a whole Pandora's box of emotions. Stop for a moment to analyse the real emotion behind your stress. Are you bored when you eat? Angry? Overwhelmed? Sad? Once you decide what's bothering you, you'll be able to find better alternatives to munching the feeling away. If you're overwhelmed, take time to get organised instead of racing for the biscuit tin. If you're sad, lie in a hot bath sprinkled with lavender while you listen to music. If you're angry, take a run or a brisk walk. For handling long-term stress, experts recommend learning meditation or deep-breathing techniques.

Old attitude: *I have no willpower. If the chocolates are there, I'm going to eat the whole box.*
New attitude: *I am an adult who can and will make rational choices about what I eat.*

Ask yourself, 'Am I making a conscious decision to eat this, or am I getting carried away by my emotions? Am I trying to avoid working, so I'm eating instead?' Once you learn to differentiate between a want and a choice you'll begin to have a much more relaxed relationship with food. A choice is rational. A want is emotional.

Think about what you crave and why, then substitute something satisfying but lower in fat and calories. When you're about to dig into the chocolate chip cookies, ask yourself if it's the crunchiness that appeals to you or the sweetness. Would a crunchy carrot dipped in fat-free dressing do? Or a cup of hot chocolate made with skimmed milk?

If you feel that you really do want a cookie, decide if you can eat just one or two. If you can't, eat more, but realise it is your choice. Your brain is not at the mercy of a rushing torrent of need. Thinking through your choice prevents out-of-control bingeing.

Old attitude: *I tried counting calories and measuring out portions for a while. But then I seemed to go mad and ate more than ever. I don't think it's possible for me to eat in moderation, especially when it comes to something like cheese and onion crisps. They're meant to be eaten by the bag in front of the TV.*

New attitude: *I'm not going to force myself to go on a rigid diet. I'm going to learn healthier ways of eating for life.*

Give portion control another try but this time use it as a guideline and not as a restriction. Measure out once those foods you like. Take a look at the fat and calorie content, so you'll have a general idea how much they add to your total food intake for the day. But don't weigh and measure everything on a daily basis or you really *will* go mad.

Old attitude: *part of food's appeal is the camaraderie. At my office, eating chocolate is a common bond among the women I work with. We talk about it, share it and give it to each other.*

New attitude: *I'm going to appreciate my friends for who they are and not what we eat together. I'm going to ask them to do the same.*

Try taking charge. What would happen if you proposed to your fellow chocolate-lovers that you all embark on a month of healthy eating?

You could still share the eating elements of your friendship without having to sacrifice something important to you – getting in shape. Buy and share unusual fruit, or make healthy packed lunches that you can all dip into.

Also, give your friends some credit. If they care about you, they'll want the best for you. Explain your reasons for wanting to make some changes and ask for their help. You may be surprised at their warm response.

Old attitude: *my mother and sister are health food nuts. I grew up having to hide my Mars bars. Even as an adult, I feel they're still pressuring me to lose weight – and now my husband*

has joined in. I was always a rebel, so my immediate reaction is to eat as much food as I can get my hands on.

New attitude: *I'm going to take responsibility for my own well-being. I need to tune them out and go about losing weight slowly and patiently in my own way.*

If you're eating to satisfy or annoy someone else you have lost touch with your inner voice, the one that will guide you to foods you enjoy while you accomplish personal goals for your body and your life. Explore your own motivations for changing your eating patterns. How do you feel when you overeat? How do you feel when you eat healthy meals all day and go for a walk? What are your personal goals for fitness and health? Value yourself and let motivation for change come from within. You may be pleasantly surprised that healthy eating is a springboard for other changes in your life.

Old attitude: *I know women who stay slim because they exercise all the time and eat lots of beans and grains. But that's not for me. I refuse to abandon all fun in my life and eat strange foods.*

New attitude: *I'm not going to eat foods I hate, but I will try new things. Making healthy lifestyle choices is fun, and doing something good for myself is satisfying.*

Who says 'strange' foods have to taste bad? You might discover that your friend eating tabbouleh does so because it's delicious!

Buy one thing you haven't tried before every time you go to the supermarket.

Beyond new choices, you may be underestimating the number of healthy foods you already like.

Every food group contains many choices. So if you hate bulgur and cottage cheese, eat wholemeal bread and a low-fat pudding instead. For other suggestions, see the 'New Foods to Try' sections throughout Part 2.

Old attitude: *I see women who can eat anything they want and still stay thin as a rail. I'm* *short, and I gain weight when I just think about food. It's not fair.*

New attitude: *I'm going to concentrate on looking and feeling my best and stop dwelling on things I can't change.*

Life is indeed unfair so start by accepting that, say experts. Your genetic background, metabolism, skeletal structure and body type all factor into the person you see when you look in the mirror. If you're destined to be a round person, you're never going to be a skinny, Twiggy-type person. You can exercise and eat healthy foods, however, to make your figure proportionate and firm. As a bonus, you can also keep your heart healthy and your bones strong.

Don't compare yourself to the slender woman eating the three-cheese pizza – you don't know how much she exercises. Maybe that's the first meal she's eaten all day, and that's not very healthy.

Old attitude: *I lost 3½ stone (25kg). Now I don't have to worry any more and I can finally eat anything I want.*

New attitude: *my new food attitude is a healthy and productive one. I can indulge in chocolate cake once in a while, but my switch to healthy eating is something I'll stick with for a lifetime.*

If you gained weight in the first place, you're prone to regaining it. The 'I'm fixed now' syndrome is the biggest reason people put it back on, no matter how thrilled they were to reach their goals.

Stick with your food diary and study it periodically to identify where you might be vulnerable. If you never really got out of the habit of munching a late-night snack, for example, make sure you're stocked up with fresh fruit or crispbread and pretzels. Sometimes it's easier to change the food than your behaviour pattern.

Personal Food Diary

Experts say the best way to get an accurate picture of what you're eating is to keep a food diary for three days. Photocopy these pages and then continue to record what you eat, including snacks and beverages. That helps you to look at your overall diet, rather than focusing on 'good' or 'bad' foods at any one meal.

Date
Breakfast
Lunch
Dinner
Snacks
Beverages

Date
Breakfast
Lunch
Dinner
Snacks
Beverages

Date
Breakfast
Lunch
Dinner
Snacks
Beverages

Personal Food Diary

Date

Breakfast

Lunch

Dinner

Snacks

Beverages

Date

Breakfast

Lunch

Dinner

Snacks

Beverages

Date

Breakfast

Lunch

Dinner

Snacks

Beverages

Date

Breakfast

Lunch

Dinner

Snacks

Beverages

Chapter 13

Action Tips
for Exercisers

So you're convinced: getting some form of calorie-burning exercise a couple of times a week is the only way you're going to leave un-wanted pounds behind. Doing crunches, leg raises and other forms of resistance training for your tummy, backside, hips and thighs is the right solution. The question is, just when is all this exercise going to take place? Finding time – and staying motivated – aren't always easy.

Problem: *you hate exercise.*
Solution: *choose activities that you truly enjoy. Just because your sister-in-law runs, your neighbour goes for marathon bike rides and your pals at the office go to aerobics classes doesn't mean you have to. Opt for something you like.*

Problem: *you've tried exercise before, but you dropped out after two or three sessions.*
Solution: *announce your intentions to your family and friends. This makes it more likely that you'll stick to your programme.*

Problem: *you exercise every day for the first week, then get distracted, and by week three you've abandoned exercise altogether.*
Solution: *start out exercising just twice a week. This leaves room for you to want to do more, instead of setting yourself up for failure because you haven't fulfilled greater ambitions.*

Problem: *you have too much to do and too little time.*

Solution: *surveys show that most people who want to exercise but don't blame lack of time. You can find the time, though. Here's how.*

- Decide on your best time of day. Some women get up early to work out first thing in the morning. Others can't function before two cups of coffee, so they save their workouts for later in the day.

- Make exercise appointments in your diary or stick a reminder on your refrigerator door. This helps you get into a habit while also training your family to anticipate and respect your exercise regimen. Fit other appointments around your exercise session, rather than vice versa.

- Do it for 10 minutes. Studies have shown that accumulating 30 minutes of daily exercise in 10-minute chunks has positive calorie-burning and heart-strengthening effects.

- Try walking 10 minutes before work, do another 10 at lunchtime and 10 minutes after dinner.

- Exercise with short videos. A number of exercise videos now incorporate a week's worth of short – no longer than 15 minutes – routines on the same tape. Do one routine a day and rewind at the end of the week.

- Walk around the block while the dinner's cooking.

- Make phone calls on a speaker or mobile phone while you're on a treadmill or bike or doing a stretch routine. In fact, this is a great time to take the 'talk test' of exercise intensity: you should be able to breathe well enough to hold up your end of a conversation.

Problem: *my family needs me. The kids fight when I'm not available, and my husband says I'm ignoring him.*
Solution: *include your family in exercise.*

- Join a health club that offers baby-sitting services or kids' activities. You get your exercise while your children get entertained.

- Do your workout during your child's sports practice. Instead of just daydreaming on the sidelines, walk, jog or bike.

- Use very small children as exercise aids. Plop your seated infant at your feet and do curl-ups towards her, saying 'peek-a-boo' as you sit up. Or sit in a chair, balance your toddler astride your ankles and shins, hold her hands, and bounce her gently up and down, working your quadriceps.

- Encourage your husband to exercise with you. This can be a big boost to your routine while relieving the guilt that can arise from 'abandoning' your spouse to do something for yourself.

- If you still have problems, talk it over with your family. Explain the changes you want to make, why they're important to you, and what help you'll need from them. For example, 'I want to go for a walk three mornings a week, so you'll need to get up and eat breakfast by yourselves.' If your plans will cause them difficulties, work out compromise solutions.

Problem: *my family doesn't seem to mind if I exercise, but I still feel guilty when I leave them in order to work out.*
Solution: *tell yourself you deserve some time to take care of your body.*

- Consider yourself a positive role model for your children. Your routine will demonstrate the benefits of exercise, from having more energy to being in a better mood. Emphasise the concept by taking your child along on walks and bike rides whenever you can.

Problem: *you work in an office all day and can't fit in any exercise.*
Solution: *be creative and flexible.*

- Arrange to have flexible working hours if you can. If you start later you can go to the gym before work; if earlier, you can exercise after work. Or extend your working day so you can take a long lunch break for exercise.

- Exercise in your office. Close the door and do crunches or push-ups. If you don't have privacy, do exercises in your chair like 'writing the alphabet' with your toes, which works your shins and calves. Trace each letter from A to Z on the floor with the big toe of each foot. You can also strengthen your thighs by tightening and releasing them while sitting.

Problem: *you work the night shift.*
Solution: *there's no rule that says you can't exercise at odd hours. As long as you're getting enough sleep and have a safe place to exercise – say, on home exercise equipment – there's no reason you can't exercise after your midnight shift.*

Problem: *you have trouble staying motivated when you exercise alone.*
Solution: *make exercise time social time.*

- When a friend asks you out to a movie or for a drink, suggest that you go for a swim together instead.

- Tell your colleagues you're going for a walk during your lunch hour, and ask them to join you.

- Get an 'exercise buddy'. Working out alone can be a welcome break, but having a commitment to work out with someone else makes it more likely you'll actually do it. Choose someone who is convenient, such as a neighbour, and who has similar exercise interests and skill levels. Agree from the outset

Quick Answers to Common Excuses

Some days, outside forces coax you to skip a workout. Should you tough it out, or ease off?

'I have period pains.' Postponing your exercise is definitely valid if you have bad menstrual cramps or heavy bleeding. But a little exercise may actually help relieve cramping. Do it for just a few minutes and see how you feel.

'I have flu.' If you're ill, hang up your trainers. Exercising now will probably only make you feel worse, especially if you have a fever. When your body is fighting a virus, it needs rest and lots of fluids to marshal its resources to fight the bug.

'It's rainy and cold outside.' Carry a mini folding umbrella with you so you don't have to miss your walk during a shower, or wear a waterproof jogging outfit. In cold weather, wrap up warmly (see page 211).

'It's too dark to exercise outside by the time I get home.' Wear white clothing and reflective gear to protect yourself in traffic when you're out in the dark. If you exercise at a gym at night and are concerned about safety, go with a friend or at least ask someone at the gym to walk you to your car after your workout.

'Business travel and holidays mess up my routine.' Sneak exercise into your travel plans. At airports, challenge yourself to walk alongside, but faster than, the travelators. At your destination, see the sights on foot. Stay at a hotel with exercise facilities, or take a skipping rope with you. Pack an exercise video and plug it into your hotel room's VCR if it has one. And consider an active holiday spent hiking, biking or skiing.

that you'll both be positive and supportive rather than critical of each other.

- Have an 'online buddy'. If you have access to the Internet, send e-mail messages about your workouts to online exercise buddies.

Problem: *you can't afford a lot of expensive equipment, gym fees or fancy workout clothes.*
Solution: *keep it simple.*

- Take up walking or jogging, or use exercise videos.
- Join a gym where you can pay per month or per session. Then go only when you need to – like when it's too cold to exercise outdoors.
- Ask for workout clothes instead of other gifts for your birthday, Christmas or other special occasions. The same goes for exercise gear like water aerobics aids, aerobic videos, a gel seat for your bike and so forth.

Problem: *you'd like to go to the gym but it's just too much trouble to drive there, especially in bad weather.*
Solution: *exercise at home.*

- A motorised treadmill, exercise bike or exercise video will do just fine for aerobic exercise. And you can do your workouts to trim your abdominals, hips, thighs and buttocks at home on a mat.
- To create the feel of a health club and help you to keep an eye on your form, install a mirror.
- Tell your family that you need some time for yourself. Unless they're going to work out with you this is your time, not the time to help your kids with their maths homework.

Problem: *your hair and make-up get messed up when you exercise, and you have to go back to work.*
Solution: *dealing with perspiration will solve both problems. Perspiration makes frizzy hair frizzier and straight hair limp. It also can cause make-up to streak.*

- Pull your hair back to get it off your neck. This will keep you cooler and your hair will be less likely to get wet, which can destroy any hairdo.

- Avoid wearing make-up during exercise. Combined with perspiration, it may irritate your skin. If you don't want to remove and reapply your makeup for a quick lunchtime workout, use the kind that doesn't run. Then, to prevent streaks, gently dab perspiration with a soft towel as you exercise.

Problem: *you mean to work out, but you forget your workout clothes half the time, or you're too rushed to get your exercise gear together before leaving for work.*
Solution: *plan ahead. Pack your workout clothes a day in advance or have extra workout clothes stashed in your desk at work.*

Problem: *you start out with enthusiasm, but you can't stay motivated.*
Solution: *remind yourself why you're doing this.*

- Put your reasons down on paper. Write down both the benefits of exercising and getting in shape and the costs of not doing so. For example, 'Benefit of exercising: I look better in my clothes. Cost of not exercising: I feel fat, tired and bad about myself.' Display your list in a prominent place.

- Mentally rehearse your exercise. What your mind believes your body achieves. When you wake up in the morning, spend a few moments in bed mentally picturing yourself exercising. Surround yourself with inspirational posters and pictures of women involved in various forms of exercise.

- Note your progress. You'll feel more motivated if you check your progress against your initial goals every two months or so.

- Train for an ambitious goal. Once you're in the swing of regular exercise, pump up your motivation by aiming for an event. For example, if you're a walker or runner, sign up for a local race.

Problem: *some days exercise feels easy, but sometimes it's a real effort to get through.*
Solution: *expect tough days and deal with them – it happens to even the most avid of exercisers. Remember that tomorrow is another day. If you are slowed by a physical rather than a mental problem, however, take it easy.*

Problem: *you react to any setback with frustration and give up.*
Solution: *backsliding is normal. Maybe your old habits caught up with you or life got so hectic that you didn't exercise for a week or two. Just get back on track as quickly as possible and don't waste time beating yourself over the head about it.*

Problem: *you've been exercising for months, but you're getting bored and you can't get excited about activities you used to enjoy.*
Solution: *these are signs that your exercise regimen is getting stale. To renew your interest:*

- Change the scenery. If you usually work out indoors, logging miles on a treadmill or exercise bike, move your workout outside. Or bring your running-around-the-block workout inside.

- Take up an entirely new activity. If you've always stuck to solitary pursuits, get involved in a team sport such as netball or a partner game such as tennis. Or sign up for a class to train for running a marathon.

- Watch television or listen to music on headphones while you're walking on a treadmill or lifting weights. For your exercise bike and stairclimber at home, buy a plastic rack that fits on to the console and holds reading material and a water bottle. Don't wear Walkman-type headphones when you're out on the road, however: you won't be able to hear traffic.

- Try an occasional maximum-effort workout: if you always do 25 crunches, aim for as many as you can without getting muscular cramp. If you jog, go to a local track and run a mile as fast as you can, timing yourself.

- Try new exercise toys. Heart rate monitors, exercise tubes and rubber bands, Swiss balls and aquatic exercise gear can make workouts more fun and challenging. Find out which new training gadgets are available for your favourite activity, or try something altogether new with them.

Personal Exercise Log

Date

The key to banishing your belly, butt and thighs with exercise is consistency. Photocopy this exercise log and use it to record your aerobic efforts and body-shaping workouts every day. You should see results in as little as four weeks!

Aerobic Exercise	
Activity	Duration

Workouts for Waist and Tummy	
Exercise	Sets/reps
Curl-Ups 1	
Curl-Ups 2	
Curl-Ups 3	
Knee-Up Crunches	
Crunches with Knees Up, Spread	
Inclined Board Crunches	
Hip Raises	
Modified Knee Raises	
Pelvic Tilts	
Reverse Curls	
Single-Knee Lifts	
Diagonal Curl-Ups 1	
Diagonal Curl-Ups 2	
Diagonal Curl-Ups 3	
Side Crunches	
Side Bends	
Side Jack-knives	

Workouts for Hips, Thighs and Buttocks	
Exercise	Sets/reps
Leg Extensions	
Lunges	
Squats	
Wall Squats	
Leg Curls	
Prone Single-Leg Raises	
Back Leg Extensions	
Bent-Leg Extensions	
Pelvic Lifts	
Bent-Knee Crossovers	
Side-Lying Straight-Leg Raises	
Standing Abductions	
Seated Abductions	
Side-Lying Bent-Leg Raises	
Fire Hydrants	
Inner Leg Raises	
Seated Inner Leg Raises	
Butterfly Leg Raises	
Single-Leg Pelvic Lifts	
Scissors	

INDEX

Page numbers in **bold** type refer to illustrations

XYZ